Respiratory Medicine
on the Move

This book provides a convenient distillation of the specialty in note form, ideal for the busy medical student and junior doctor. No matter what your learning style, whether you are studying the subject for the first time or revisiting it during exam preparation, **Respiratory Medicine on the Move** is structured to deliver the right information whenever and wherever you need it.

Dip into the book as needed for information to suit different clinical and learning situations and you really will learn medicine on the move!

Medicine on the Move

Editor-in-chief: Rory Mackinnon
Series editors: Sally Keat, Thomas Locke,
Andrew Walker and Harriet Walker

Obstetrics, Gynaecology and Women's Health on the Move
Amie Clifford, Claire Kelly, Chris Yau and Sally Hallam, 2012

Orthopaedics and Rheumatology on the Move
Terence McLoughlin, Ian Baxter and Nicole Abdul, 2013

Surgery on the Move
Jenna Morgan, Harriet Walker and Andrew Viggars, 2014

Neurology and Clinical Neuroanatomy on the Move
Matthew Tate, Johnathan Cooper-Knock, Zoe Hunter and Elizabeth Wood, 2014

Gastroenterology on the Move
Arash Assadsangabi, Lucy Carroll and Andrew Irvine, 2015

Emergency and Acute Medicine on the Move
Naomi Meardon, Shireen Siddiqui, Elena Del Vescovo, Lucy C Peart and Sherif Hemaya, 2015

Cardiology and the Cardiovascular System on the Move
David Dunleavy, Swati Gupta and Alexandra Marsh, 2015

Clinical Pharmacology and Practical Prescribing on the Move
James Turnbull and Matthew Tate, 2016

Respiratory Medicine on the Move
Isabelle van Heeswijk and Michael Naughton, 2024

More details can be found at https://www.routledge.com/Medicine-on-the-Move/book-series/CRCMEDIONMOV - Routledge & CRC Press

Respiratory Medicine
on the Move

Authors: **Isabelle van Heeswijk**
and Michael Naughton
Editorial Advisor: **Paul Beckett**

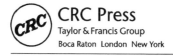

CRC Press
Taylor & Francis Group
Boca Raton London New York

CRC Press is an imprint of the
Taylor & Francis Group, an **informa** business

Designed cover image: Shutterstock

First edition published 2025
by CRC Press
2385 NW Executive Center Drive, Suite 320, Boca Raton FL 33431

and by CRC Press
4 Park Square, Milton Park, Abingdon, Oxon, OX14 4RN

CRC Press is an imprint of Taylor & Francis Group, LLC

© 2025 Isabelle van Heeswijk and Michael Naughton

ISBN: 978-1-032-77937-9 (hbk)
ISBN: 978-1-498-72770-9 (pbk)
ISBN: 978-1-315-11393-7 (ebk)

DOI: 10.1201/9781315113937

Typeset in Adobe Garamond Pro
by Apex CoVantage, LLC

Contents

Abbreviations

- 6MWT: 6-minute walk test
- ABG: Arterial blood gas
- ABPA: Allergic bronchopulmonary aspergillosis
- ACE: Angiotensin converting enzyme
- ADH: Anti-diuretic hormone
- AFB: Acid-fast bacillus
- AFP: Alpha fetoprotein
- AHI: Apnoea-hypopnoea index
- AIDS: Acquired immune deficiency syndrome
- AIP: Acute interstitial pneumonia
- AIS: Adenocarcinoma in situ
- ANA: Antinuclear antibody
- ANCA: Anti-neutrophil cytoplasmic antibody
- ANP: Atrial natriuretic peptide
- AP: Anteroposterior
- APTT: Activated partial thromboplastin time
- APUD: Amine precursor uptake and decarboxylation
- ARDS: Acute respiratory distress syndrome
- AV: Arterio-venous
- BAC: Bronchoalveolar carcinoma
- BAL: Bronchoalveolar lavage
- BCG: Bacillus Calmette-Guérin
- BD: Twice daily
- BDP: Beclometasone diproprionate
- BiPAP: Bilevel positive airway pressure
- BMI: Body mass index
- BNP: Brain natriuretic peptide
- BODE: BMI, obstruction, dyspnoea, exercise capacity
- BP: Blood pressure
- BTS: British Thoracic Society
- cANCA: Cytoplasmic anti-neutrophil cytoplasmic antibody
- CAP: Community-acquired pneumonia
- CF: Cystic fibrosis
- CFRD: Cystic fibrosis–related diabetes
- CFTR: Cystic fibrosis transmembrane conductance regulator
- CMV: Cytomegalovirus
- CNS: Central nervous system
- COP: Cryptogenic organising pneumonia
- COPD: Chronic obstructive pulmonary disease
- CPAP: Continuous positive airway pressure

Abbreviations

- CRP: C-reactive protein
- CSS: Churg-Strauss syndrome
- CT: Computerised tomography
- CTEPH: Chronic thromboembolic pulmonary hypertension
- CTPA: Computerised tomography pulmonary angiogram
- CURB-65: Confusion, urea, respiratory rate, blood pressure, 65
- CXR: Chest X-ray
- DIP: Desquamative interstitial pneumonia
- DOTS: Directly observed treatment, short course
- DVT: Deep vein thrombosis
- EBUS: Endobronchial ultrasound
- ECG: Electrocardiogram
- ED: Emergency Department
- EEG: Electroencephalogram
- EGFR-TK: Epidermal growth factor receptor tyrosine kinase
- EGPA: Eosinophilic granulomatosis with polyangiitis
- EIA: Enzyme immunoassay
- EPTB: Extra-pulmonary tuberculosis
- ESRD: End-stage renal disease
- ESS: Epworth Sleepiness Scale
- FBC: Full blood count
- FeNO: Fractional exhaled nitric oxide
- FEV1: Forced expiratory volume in 1 second
- FEV1/FVC: Forced expiratory volume in 1 second/forced vital capacity rati·
- FVC: Forced vital capacity
- GBM: Glomerular basement membrane
- GCT: Germ cell tumour
- GORD: Gastro-oesophageal reflux disease
- GPA: Granulomatosis with polyangiitis (Wegener's granulomatosis)
- GPS: Goodpasture's syndrome
- H: Haemagglutinin
- HAART: Highly active antiretroviral therapy
- HAP: Hospital-acquired pneumonia
- HGV: Heavy goods vehicle
- HIV: Human immunodeficiency virus
- HRCT: High-resolution computerised tomography
- IA: Inflammatory arthritis
- ICSI: Intracytoplasmic sperm injection
- ICU: Intensive care unit
- IgE: Immunoglobulin E
- IgG: Immunoglobulin G
- IGRA: Interferon gamma release assays
- ILD: Interstitial lung disease
- INR: International normalised ratio

- IPAH: Idiopathic pulmonary arterial hypertension
- IPF: Idiopathic pulmonary fibrosis
- IRIS: Immune reconstitution inflammatory syndrome
- IV: Intravenous
- IVC: Inferior vena cava
- JVP: Jugular venous pressure
- KUB: Kidney, ureter, bladder
- LABA: Long-acting beta agonist
- LDH: Lactate dehydrogenase
- LFTs: Liver function tests
- LIP: Lymphoid interstitial pneumonia
- LMWH: Low-molecular-weight heparin
- LRTI: Lower respiratory tract infection
- LTOT: Long-term oxygen therapy
- LV: Left ventricle
- MAC: Mycobacterium avium complex
- MAD: Mandibular advancement device
- MALT: Mucosa-associated lymphoid tissue
- MC&S: Microscopy, culture and sensitivity
- MDR-TB: Multidrug-resistant tuberculosis
- MGIT: Mycobacteria growth indicator tube
- MPA: Microscopic polyangiitis
- MRSA: Methicillin-resistant Staphylococcus aureus
- N: Neuraminidase
- NICE: National Institute for Health and Care Excellence
- NIV: Non-invasive ventilation
- NPPV: Non-invasive positive pressure ventilation
- NRT: Nicotine replacement therapy
- NSAID: Non-steroidal anti-inflammatory drug
- NSCLC: Non–small cell lung cancer
- NSIP: Non-specific interstitial pneumonia
- NTM: Non-tuberculous mycobacteria
- ODI: Oxygen desaturation index
- OSAHS: Obstructive sleep apnoea/hypopnea syndrome
- PA: Posteroanterior
- PaCO2: Partial pressure of carbon dioxide in arterial blood
- PAH: Pulmonary arterial hypertension
- pANCA: Perinuclear anti-neutrophil cytoplasmic antibody
- PaO2: Partial pressure of oxygen in arterial blood
- PCD: Primary ciliary dyskinesia
- PCP: Pneumocystis jirovecii pneumonia
- PCR: Polymerase chain reaction
- PE: Pulmonary embolism
- PEF: Peak expiratory flow

- PEFR: Peak expiratory flow rate
- PEP: Positive expiratory pressure
- PFT: Pulmonary function test
- PO: Per os (orally)
- PPE: Personal protective equipment
- PPI: Proton pump inhibitor
- PR3: Proteinase 3
- PSG: Polysomnography
- PSP: Primary spontaneous pneumothorax
- PVR: Peripheral vascular resistance
- QDS: Four times daily
- QoL: Quality of life
- RB-ILD: Respiratory bronchiolitis–associated interstitial lung disease
- RCP: Royal College of Physicians
- RV: Right ventricle
- SABA: Short-acting beta agonist
- SBOT: Short burst oxygen therapy
- SBP: Systolic blood pressure
- SCLC: Small cell lung cancer
- SIADH: Syndrome of inappropriate antidiuretic hormone secretion
- SLE: Systemic lupus erythematosus
- SSP: Secondary spontaneous pneumothorax
- SVC: Superior vena cava
- SVCO: Superior vena cava obstruction
- TB: Tuberculosis
- TDS: Three times daily
- TFTs: Thyroid function tests
- Tlco: Transfer factor for carbon monoxide
- TNF: Tumour necrosis factor
- TST: Tuberculin skin test
- TTE: Transthoracic echocardiogram
- U&E: Urea and electrolytes
- UFH: Unfractionated heparin
- UIP: Usual interstitial pneumonia
- URTI: Upper respiratory tract infection
- USS: Ultrasound scan
- V/Q scan: Ventilation/perfusion scan
- VATS: Video-assisted thoracoscopic surgery
- VC: Vital capacity
- WCC: White cell count
- WHO: World Health Organisation
- XDR-TB: Extensively drug-resistant tuberculosis

An Explanation of the Text

The book is divided into two parts covering the clinical aspects of respiratory medicine, including investigations and prescribing, and a self-assessment section. We have used bullet points to keep the text concise and supplemented this with a range of diagrams, pictures and MICRO boxes (explained below).

Where possible we have endeavoured to include treatment options for the conditions covered. Nevertheless, drug sensitivities and clinical practices are constantly under review, so always check your local guidelines for up-to-date information.

You will find the following resources useful to find out more about any of the drugs mentioned in this book:

BNF (at www.bnf.org/bnf/index.htm)

eMC (at www.medicines.org.uk/emc/)

MICRO-facts

These boxes expand on the text and contain clinically relevant facts and memorable summaries of the essential information.

MICRO-print

These boxes contain additional information to the text that may interest certain readers but is not essential for everybody to learn.

MICRO-case

These boxes contain clinical cases relevant to the text and include a number of summary bullet points to highlight the key learning objectives.

MICRO-references

These boxes contain references to important clinical research and national guidance.

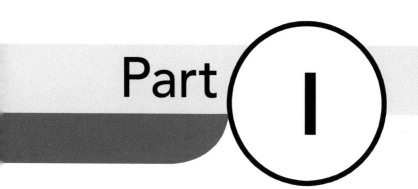

Part I

Respiratory Medicine

1 Clinical Assessment

1.1 HISTORY

1. HISTORY OF PRESENTING COMPLAINT

- **Breathlessness:**
    - **Onset:** sudden or gradual?
    - **Timing:** on exercise or at rest?
        - If shortness of breath on exertion, clarify the patient's exercise tolerance. "How far can you walk before you have to stop because of your breathing?"
        - Compare this to their "normal" exercise tolerance or tolerance before this episode of breathlessness.
    - **Timing:** nocturnal/early morning symptoms?
    - **Duration.**
    - **Exacerbating factors:** cold air, exercise, dust, pets, drugs.
    - **Relieving factors:** medications, rest.
    - **Severity – the MRC Dyspnoea Scale can be used (see** Table 1.1)
    - **Orthopnoea or paroxysmal nocturnal dyspnoea?**
        - These are suggestive of cardiac failure.
    - **Other features.**

Table 1.1 **MRC Dyspnoea Scale.**

DESCRIPTION	GRADE
I only get breathless with strenuous exercise	0
I get short of breath when hurrying on level ground or walking up a slight hill	1
On level ground, I walk slower than people of my age because of breathlessness, or I have to stop for breath when walking at my own pace on the level	2
I stop for breath after walking about 100 yards or after a few minutes on level ground	3
I am too breathless to leave the house or I am breathless when dressing/undressing	4

DOI: 10.1201/9781315113937-2

- **Cough:**
    - **Onset:** acute or chronic?
    - **Diurnal variability:** overnight/early morning suggests asthma.
    - **Exacerbating factors.**
    - **Productive or unproductive?**
        - **If productive, ask about sputum:**
            - **Colour:** see Table 1.2.
            - **Consistency:** see Table 1.2.
            - **Quantity:** large quantities are associated with bronchiectasis.
            - **Odour:** foul-smelling or foul-tasting sputum suggests anaerobic infection.
            - **Presence or absence of blood.**

Table 1.2 **Characteristic sputum appearances in respiratory disease.**

SPUTUM TYPE	COLOUR	CONSISTENCY	CAUSE
Serous	Clear/Pink	Thin Watery/Frothy	Acute – pulmonary oedema Chronic – alveolar cancer
Mucoid	Clear/White/ Grey	Viscid	COPD Asthma
Purulent	Yellow	Thick	Acute infection Asthma
	Green	Thick	Chronic infection: Pneumonia Bronchiectasis Cystic fibrosis Lung abscess
Rusty	Rusty Red	Thick	Pneumococcal pneumonia

- **Haemoptysis:**
    - Clarify if fresh blood e.g. bright red or dark altered blood.
    - If mixed with sputum, this may reflect an infective aetiology, but this is not exclusive.
    - Volume >200 mL in 24 hours is considered "massive haemoptysis" (see Chapter 18: Respiratory Emergencies).
    - Pure red blood may reflect a bleed from a bronchial artery (as in bronchiectasis, pulmonary emboli and malignancy).
    - Any features of vasculitis? (Patient may have alveolar haemorrhage; see Chapter 13: Vasculitis and the lung.)

- **Pain:**
  - **Pleuritic pain:** sharp, stabbing, worse on inspiration.
    - Causes include pulmonary embolism (PE), pneumonia, pneumothorax, rib fracture, musculoskeletal pain.
  - **Chest wall pain:**
    - **Localised, following trauma:** rib fracture or muscular strain.
    - **Dermatomal:** herpes zoster.
    - **Progressive dull, aching, gnawing pain:** consider malignancy.
  - **Central chest pain may be due to non-respiratory causes:**
    - **Cardiac:** central, crushing pain.
    - **Upper gastrointestinal:** associated with gastrointestinal symptoms, burning, retrosternal pain e.g. gastro-oesophageal reflux. Can be confused with aortic dissection.
    - **Aortic:** tearing pain in aortic dissection, radiates to the back.
    - **Mediastinal:** central, retrosternal and unrelated to coughing/respiration. Causes include lymphadenopathy and thymoma.

MICRO-facts

"SOCRATES": Questions to ask when enquiring about pain:

Site
Onset
Character
Radiation
Associated symptoms
Timing
Exacerbating/relieving factors
Severity.

PAST MEDICAL HISTORY

Previous atopic disease: eczema and hay fever are associated with asthma.
Recent trauma/surgery: especially useful if a PE is suspected.
Immunosuppression: increases risk of TB and atypical infection.
Perinatal illness: potential chronic lung disease of the newborn if history of prematurity, assisted delivery or admission to the neonatal unit.

DRUG HISTORY

Current inhaler use: type, dosage, frequency.
Home oxygen therapy: long-term oxygen therapy (LTOT), ambulatory or short burst oxygen therapy (SBOT).
Home nebulisers.

Respiratory Medicine

- **Long-term antibiotics for prophylaxis in COPD/bronchiectasis (usually azithromycin).**
- **Previous prescriptions for this condition.**
- **Immunosuppressive medications:** e.g. oral corticosteroid use.
- Bone protection if on regular corticosteroids e.g. calcium/vitamin D combination +/– oral bisphosphonate.
- **Anticoagulant/antiplatelet drugs:** may influence safety of procedures or biopsies.

MICRO-facts

Medications that can cause/worsen respiratory symptoms:

ACE inhibitor: causes cough due to lack of degradation of bradykinin.

Amiodarone, methotrexate, nitrofurantoin: can cause pulmonary fibrosis.

β-blockers: may worsen bronchoconstriction due to blockade of β2-adrenoceptors in the lungs.

Non-steroidal anti-inflammatory drugs: may cause bronchospasm in asthmatics due to an increase in leukotriene production.

---

4. ALLERGIES

- Ask about drug allergies before prescribing any drug.
- Relevant if anaphylaxis is suspected.
- Allergic/atopic disease is associated with asthma.

5. FAMILY HISTORY

- **Genetic diseases:** cystic fibrosis, α1-antitrypsin deficiency.
- **Atopic diseases:** eczema, hay fever, asthma.
- **Venous thromboembolism (VTE):** may suggest a familial thrombophilia.
- **Malignancy:** although 50% of people born after 1960 will be diagnosed with some form of cancer in their lifetime (https://cancerresearchuk.org), th lacks specificity.
- **History of TB in the family.**

6. SOCIAL HISTORY

- **Smoking history:** see MICRO-Facts (below).
- **Inhaled drugs.**
- **Housing:** overcrowding is a risk factor for TB and infection.
- **Pets:**
    - **Cats, dogs, rodents:** may worsen atopic disease.
    - **Birds:** associated with hypersensitivity pneumonitis and psittacosis pneumonia.

MICRO-facts

Calculating "pack-years"
Pack-years = (number of cigarettes smoked per day) × (number of years smoked)/20.

OCCUPATION

Asbestos exposure: in shipyards, building, plumbing and family members washing asbestos-covered work clothes (see Chapter 17: Occupational lung disease).
Dust exposure: silicon, coal dust, flour.
Occupational asthma (see Chapter 17: Occupational lung disease for high-risk occupations).

TRAVEL HISTORY

Any travel to TB endemic regions? How long ago?
Any other travel: may increase risk of atypical infection.

1.2 EXAMINATION

GENERAL INSPECTION

Around the bed area: inhalers, oxygen, nebuliser, sputum pot, CPAP or NIV machine.
Of the patient: colour, comfort, nutritional status and respiratory rate.
Signs of respiratory distress:
- Pursed-lip breathing.
- Use of accessory muscles.
- High respiratory rate (>20 breaths/min).
- Cyanosis (central or peripheral).
- Difficulty completing sentences.

HANDS

Clubbing: loss of angle between nail and nail bed, increased nail bed fluctuance (feels spongy), increased curvature of nail and increased soft tissue bulk over terminal phalanx (Figure 1.1).

Respiratory Medicine

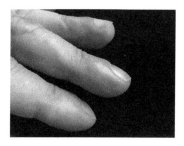 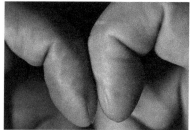

Figure 1.1 A patient with clubbing of fingernails.

MICRO-facts

Respiratory causes of clubbing – "BE CALM":

Bronchiectasis
Empyema
Cystic fibrosis
Abscess
Lung fibrosis
Malignancy.

- **Tar staining:** yellow/brown staining seen in smokers.
- **Muscle wasting:**
  - Generalised wasting/cachexia associated with emphysema or malignancy.
  - Focal wasting of intrinsic muscles between thumb and first finger due to compression of the medial cord of the brachial plexus (T1 root) by apical lung cancer.
- **Tremor:** fine tremor from β-agonist use.
- **Asterixis:** flapping tremor of CO_2 retention when wrist extended at 90 degrees.
- **Purpura and muscle wasting in limbs:** long-term or frequent corticosteroid use.

3. FACE

- **Central cyanosis (Figure 1.2).**
- **Horner's syndrome:** miosis, ptosis and anhidrosis associated with Pancoast's (apical) tumour.
- **Facial swelling:** from superior vena cava obstruction.
- **Moon-like facies:** Cushing's syndrome precipitated by long-term or frequent corticosteroid use.
- **Poor dentition:** risk factor for lung abscess.

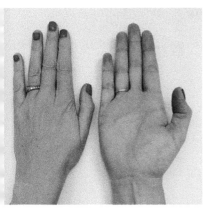
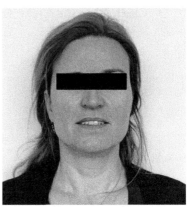

Figure 1.2 A patient with central cyanosis, showing classic bluish discolouration of lips.

NECK

- **Inspect for raised jugular venous pressure (JVP):** seen in right heart failure (pulsatile) and superior vena cava obstruction (non-pulsatile).
- **Palpate the cervical lymph nodes.**
- **Palpate for tracheal deviation:** the trachea will deviate towards a collapsed lung and away from a tension pneumothorax or massive effusion.

PRECORDIUM

- **Palpate the apex beat:** deviation occurs in tension pneumothorax.
- **Auscultate.**

CHEST

- **Inspection:**
  - Scars
  - Symmetry
  - Shape:
    - **Pectus carinatum (pigeon chest):**
      - Protrusion of the sternum and adjacent costal cartilages.
      - Accompanied by rib indrawing.
      - Historically associated with rickets.
      - May be seen in severe childhood asthma.
    - **Pectus excavatum (funnel chest):**
      - A congenital abnormality causing localised depression of the lower end of the sternum.
  - Muscle wasting
- **Palpation:**
  - **Assess chest expansion:** Is it restricted? Does the chest expand symmetrically?

- **Check for tactile vocal fremitus:** palpate as the patient says "ninety-nine".
  - Transmission is increased in consolidation and decreased with effusion or pneumothorax.
- **Percussion:**
  - **Resonant:** normal.
  - **Hyperresonant:** pneumothorax if unilateral; emphysema if bilateral.
  - **Dull:** consolidation, collapse and fibrosis.
  - **Stony dull:** effusion, empyema.
- **Auscultation:**
  - Listen for air entry throughout the lung fields. Is it reduced?
  - **Are breath sounds:**
    - **Vesicular?** normal "rustling" breath sounds.
    - **Bronchial?** high-pitched "hollow" or "blowing" breath sounds. Similar sound quality to listening over the trachea during normal breathing.
      - The most common cause is consolidation e.g. pneumonia.
  - **Any added breath sounds?**
    - **Wheeze:** musical sound caused by airway narrowing.
    - Usually expiratory.
      - Inspiratory when narrowing is severe.
      - Associated with asthma and COPD.
    - **Stridor:** harsh, rasping inspiratory sound caused by upper airways obstruction.
    - **Crepitations (crackles):** interrupted non-musical sounds mostly occurring during inspiration similar to opening of hook-and-loop closures.
      - Airways collapse on expiration and abruptly open during inspiration, causing a cracking noise.
      - Typically, fibrosis causes fine end-inspiratory crackles.
      - Bronchiectasis causes coarse biphasic crackles.
      - Coarse crackles (ruttles) are caused by secretions within the large airways.
      - Crackles may also occur in pulmonary oedema.
    - **Pleural rub:** creaking sound caused by the movement of inflamed parietal or visceral pleural over each other.
      - Described as the sound heard when a foot presses into snow.
  - **Assess for any change in the character of the sounds after coughing:** a change suggests the cause is bronchial secretions.
  - **Assess vocal resonance:** ask the patient to say "ninety-nine" while you auscultate.
    - Sounds are transmitted more easily across consolidation (louder) and less easily across pneumothorax, collapse or effusion (quieter).

Respiratory Medicine

7. COMPLETING THE EXAMINATION

- **Examine the legs:**
  - For deep vein thrombosis if pulmonary embolism is suspected.
  - For pedal oedema if cor pulmonale (see MICRO-Print) is suspected.
- **Examine the sputum pot.**
- **Check oxygen saturation and temperature chart.**
- **Take blood pressure.**

MICRO-print

Cor Pulmonale

"Cor pulmonale" is a term used to describe impaired right ventricular function caused by increased vascular resistance in the pulmonary circulation.

It is caused by chronic lung disease, e.g. COPD.

1.3 INVESTIGATIONS IN RESPIRATORY MEDICINE

1. CHEST X-RAY (CXR)

- One of the most commonly requested imaging investigations.
- This is produced by the projection of X-rays through the patient onto a radiographic plate.
- Differential absorption of X-rays by tissues of different densities results in five main "shades" on a black-and-white scale (Table 1.3).

Table 1.3 **Appearances on CXR.**

STRUCTURE	SHADE
Bone/calcified structures	White
Soft tissue	Grey
Fat	Dark grey
Gas	Black
Man-made structures/artifact	Bright white

Respiratory Medicine

Lung lobes

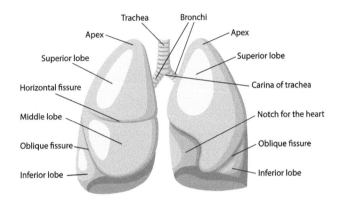

Lung segments

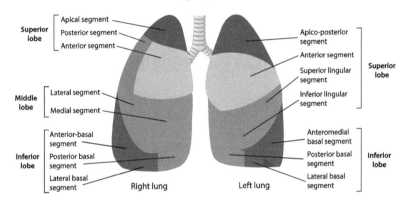

Figure 1.3 The anatomy of the lung, showing the lobe of the lung and fissures.

- **Structures that are identifiable in the lungs include:**
  - Blood vessels
  - Interlobular fissures
  - Walls of larger bronchioles.
- The lung hila should be visible bilaterally.
- Lung lobes are identifiable (see Figure 1.3).
- **NB: CXR appearances are covered with each condition throughout the book.**

2. ULTRASOUND

- Ultrasound waves are produced by passing electrical current through a piezo-electric crystal and emitted via a probe.

- The same probe detects the waves as they are reflected back by the tissues.
- The relative echogenicity of tissues are represented by shades of grey.
- In respiratory medicine, the principle uses of ultrasound are:
  - To assess the pleural space e.g. for effusions and pleural thickening.
  - For radiologically guided interventions e.g. chest drain insertion, pleural aspirations and pleural biopsies.

3. COMPUTED TOMOGRAPHY (CT)

- CT uses a rotating X-ray tube and a row of detectors to measure X-ray attenuations by different tissues inside the body.
- The data is reconstructed to produce a tomographic (cross-sectional) stack of 2D images that can be reformatted in different planes, e.g. sagittal, coronal, axial.
- Attenuation by tissue is represented by a greyscale.
  - Denser material appears brighter.
- **Volume CT with contrast:** also used in diagnosis of bronchial carcinoma, pulmonary metastases and for assessment of pneumonia complications.
- **CT pulmonary angiography (CTPA):** used to identify pulmonary embolism.
- **High-resolution CT scans (HRCT):** used to detect parenchymal lung change, e.g. bronchiectasis and pulmonary fibrosis. High-resolution doesn't mean "better", and the lack of contrast limits their utility to these conditions.
- Interpretation of chest CT is usually performed by specialists.

4. ABG

- **PaO_2: <8 kPa – hypoxaemia**
  - Always analyse PaO_2 with reference to the inspired FiO_2.
  - PaO_2 should be roughly 10kPa lower than inspired FiO_2 with normal lung function.
    - e.g. if FiO_2 is 40%, PaO_2 should be ~30 kPa.
- **$PaCO_2$ >6.5 kPa – hypercapnia**
  - $PaCO_2$ is a measure of ventilation.
  - High $PaCO_2$ in combination with low PaO_2 indicates type II respiratory failure.
  - CO_2 is an acidic gas and so any respiratory condition causing raised levels will cause a respiratory acidosis.
    - If acute, the pH will be low, but if chronic there will be renal compensation with a normal pH and a raised bicarbonate and base excess.
- **Acid-base status (Table 1.4)**

Respiratory Medicine

Respiratory Medicine

Table 1.4 Identifying acid-base disturbances.

COMPLAINT	PH	CO_2	HCO_3^-	COMMON CAUSES	COMMENTS
Respiratory acidosis	↓	↑	↑	**Acute respiratory failure:** • Life-threatening asthma • COPD exacerbation • Pneumonia **Inadequate ventilation:** • Chest wall abnormality such as severe scoliosis • Obesity hypoventilation syndrome • Neuromuscular disease • Central depression of respiration (e.g. opiates)	Elevation of HCO_3^- occurs in late phase and may be chronically raised in COPD with established respiratory failure.
Respiratory alkalosis	↑	↓	↓	Hyperventilation e.g. in anxiety or pulmonary embolism	
Metabolic acidosis	↓	↓	↓	Increased production of organic acids Increased loss of bicarbonate	Compensatory hyperventilation leads to a fall in pCO_2 which will (at least partially) offset the acidosis.
Metabolic alkalosis	↑	↑	↑	Loss of H^+ e.g. vomiting Loss of K+ e.g. diuretic use, hyperaldosteronism	Rise in pCO_2 is gradual and will plateau.

5. PULMONARY FUNCTION TESTS

- **Peak expiratory flow rate (PEFR):**
  - This is a simple bedside test that is performed by inhaling to total lung capacity then rapidly exhaling into the peak flow meter.
  - PEFR is measured in litres per minute (L/min).
  - It is most useful in the diagnosis and monitoring of asthma.
  - Typically, PEFR will be reduced in asthmatics, exhibit diurnal variability and improve in response to bronchodilator treatment.
  - Occupational asthma can be associated with an improvement in PEFR measurements when away from the workplace (weekends and holidays).
- **Spirometry:**
  - Lung volumes are measured by inhaling to total lung capacity and then fully exhaling into the spirometer (Table 1.5). The key values are:
    - **Forced expiratory volume in 1 second (FEV$_1$):** the volume of air that is exhaled in the first second of expiration.
    - **Forced vital capacity (FVC):** the total volume of air expired.
    - **Ratio of FEV$_1$/FVC.**

Table 1.5 **Spirometry findings in respiratory disease.**

PATTERN OF RESPIRATORY DISEASE	FEV$_1$	FVC	FEV$_1$/FVC	COMMON CAUSES
Obstructive	↓	↑/↔	<0.7	• Asthma • COPD
Restrictive	↓	↓↓	>0.8	Interstitial lung disease such as idiopathic pulmonary fibrosis and hypersensitivity pneumonitis Extra-thoracic lung restriction such as obesity, kyphoscoliosis and neuromuscular diseases

- **Flow-volume loop:**
  - A plot of inspiratory and expiratory flow (y-axis) against lung volumes (x-axis).
  - On expiration in normal individuals: initially there is a rapid rise in flow to the peak flow, due to:
    - Greater elastic traction of alveolar septa on airway at the beginning of expiration.
    - Greater expiratory muscle strength at the beginning of expiration.
    - Lower airway resistance initially.
  - A near linear fall in flow rate occurs with continued expiration.

Respiratory Medicine

- The inspiratory curve is a relatively symmetrical, saddle-shaped curve.
- **Abnormalities of the flow-volume loop:**
  - **Obstructive** (Figure 1.4 - see above for causes).

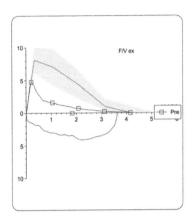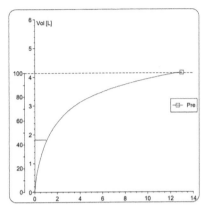

Figure 1.4 A flow volume loop from spirometry that shows obstructive lung disease.

  - **Restrictive** (Figure 1.5 - see above for causes).

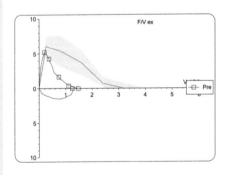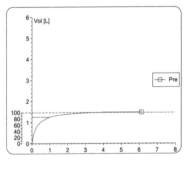

Figure 1.5 A flow volume loop from spirometry that shows restrictive lung disease.

- **Lung volumes:**
  - Can be measured using helium dilution, as helium is non-absorbable.
  - This may be inaccurate if large cystic spaces are present as helium cannot diffuse into them. In this case a body plethysmograph may be used.
  - Volumes measured include:
    - **Total lung capacity:** volume in lungs after maximal inspiration.
    - **Tidal volume:** volume of air inspired and expired during normal breathing (around 500 mL).
    - **Inspiratory reserve volume:** additional volume of air that can be inspired from the normal end-inspiratory level.

- **Functional residual capacity:** volume of air remaining in the lungs following normal expiration.
- **Vital capacity:** volume of air expired after maximal inspiration.
- **Residual volume:** volume of air remaining in lungs after maximal expiration.

- Lung volumes can also be measured by plethysmography ("body-box"), which can account for cystic spaces in the chest, but the measurement of total lung capacity includes gas elsewhere in the body (e.g. abdomen).

Transfer factor:

- The transfer factor of the lung for carbon monoxide (T_{LCO}) measures the ease with which carbon monoxide diffuses from the alveolus to capillary blood.
- The difference in partial pressure between inspired and expired carbon monoxide is measured.
  - Carbon monoxide is used for the test because it binds irreversibly to haemoglobin and therefore can be considered to move in only one direction (alveolus to blood), making the calculations much simpler.
- Anything that hinders gas transfer will reduce T_{LCO}. This includes respiratory disease, extra-thoracic restriction (such as obesity and neuromuscular diseases) and disorders affecting erythrocytes (e.g. anaemia). Blood in the airways can artificially cause an elevation of T_{LCO}.

MICRO-facts

Causes of $\downarrow T_{LCO}$:

Interstitial lung disease: fibrosis, alveolitis
Decreased lung area: restrictive diseases
Decreased perfusion: pulmonary embolism, pulmonary oedema, anaemia (the typical case is reduced TLCO with normal spirometry).

MICRO-print

During the transfer factor test a measurement of lung volume is made (the alveolar volume V_A). A "corrected" transfer factor (kCO) can be calculated by deriving T_{LCO}/V_A, and all of these will normally be included in the report.

Taking pneumonectomy as an example, the T_{LCO} is reduced because there is now only one lung, but that lung can exchange gas normally so the kCO will be normal (in fact it can even be a bit higher than normal because the one lung now gets all the cardiac output).

Similar findings are seen in conditions with extra-thoracic restriction.

Respiratory Medicine

- **Bronchodilator reversibility:**
  - Response to bronchodilators is used to distinguish between asthma and COPD when an obstructive pattern has been identified.
  - A >200 mL or >15% increase in FEV_1 from baseline favours a diagnosis of asthma.
  - An increase in FEV_1 >400 mL is strong evidence to diagnose asthma rather than COPD, although as with any test the clinical context is important.

6. BRONCHOSCOPY AND ENDOBRONCHIAL ULTRASOUND

- **Bronchoscopy:**
  - Uses a flexible scope with a video camera at the tip (allowing visualisation of the airways) as well as a working channel for suction and passage of instruments to facilitate collection of tissue samples.
  - Typically performed under local anaesthesia and light sedation.
  - It can also be used therapeutically e.g. for removal of obstructing foreign bodies and secretions; for stent insertion; and for laser resection of tumours and strictures.
    - However, these procedures are more commonly carried out by rigid bronchoscopy (under general anaesthesia) with the advantage of a wider diameter allowing larger instruments and better suction.
- **Endobronchial ultrasound (EBUS)**
  - Uses a flexible scope that houses an ultrasound probe as well as a video camera. It is mainly used to sample the hilar and mediastinal lymph nodes. Indications include:
    - Diagnosis and/or staging of thoracic malignancy.
    - Diagnosis of sarcoidosis and tuberculosis.

7. THORACOSCOPY

- An endoscopic technique used to visualise the lungs, pleura and mediastinum.
- Medical thoracoscopy is carried out using local anaesthesia and light sedation and is predominantly used to diagnose and manage pleural effusions, especially when malignancy is suspected.
- This technique is also used under general anaesthesia (video-assisted thoracoscopic surgery [VATS]) for more therapeutic purposes e.g. lobar resection, bullectomy, adhesiolysis associated with empyema and malignant disease.

8. SLEEP STUDIES

- Used in the diagnosis of obstructive sleep apnoea/hypopnea syndrome (OSAHS; see Chapter 16: Obstructive sleep apnoea).

Respiratory Medicine

Simple overnight pulse oximetry measures oxygen levels and heart rate allowing detection of desaturations and arousals. It can provide mean oxygen levels and oxygen desaturation index (ODI):

- >10 events per hour suggest OSAHS.

More detailed analysis (limited sleep study) measures a number of additional channels of information such as snore volume, nasal airflow and sleeping position.

- This allows recognition of apnoeas or hypopnoeas that don't necessarily cause enough desaturation to be picked up by oximetry alone.
- The apnoea/hypopnoea index (AHI) is calculated by summing the number of apnoeas and hypopnoeas and dividing by the number of hours of sleep.

The gold standard test is polysomnography, which adds EEG recording to the limited sleep study allowing recognition of the different phases of the sleep-wake cycle.

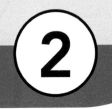

Respiratory Infection

2.1 UPPER RESPIRATORY TRACT INFECTIONS (URTIs)

- Also known as acute coryza or "the common cold".

1. DEFINITION

- Acute viral illness caused by infection with a rhinovirus.
    - Other viruses (e.g. coronavirus, influenza virus, adenovirus) sometimes implicated.

2. EPIDEMIOLOGY

- Adults may have an average of 2–4 colds per year.
- Annual epidemics occur during the winter months.

3. AETIOLOGY AND RISK FACTORS

- Spread by inhalation of respiratory droplets from infected individuals.
- Viral spread is facilitated by overcrowding and poor ventilation.

4. CLINICAL FEATURES

- **Symptoms:**
    - Nasal discharge
    - Nasal obstruction
    - Sore throat
    - Headache
    - Cough
    - Hoarseness
    - Loss of taste/smell
    - Pressure in ears/sinuses.
- **Signs:**
    - Pyrexia

5. INVESTIGATIONS

- Clinical diagnosis

DOI: 10.1201/9781315113937-3

. MANAGEMENT

- Ensure adequate fluid intake
- **Symptomatic relief:**
  - Antipyretics: ibuprofen, paracetamol, aspirin (avoid in children).
  - Analgesia: as above.
  - Decongestants: e.g. ephedrine, oxymetazoline, pseudoephedrine.
  - Cough mixtures: over-the-counter formulations, or simple honey and lemon may help alleviate symptoms.
- **Prevention:**
  - Handwashing.
  - Avoid close contact with symptomatic individuals.

2.2 INFLUENZA

. DEFINITION

An acute respiratory illness caused by the influenza virus.

. EPIDEMIOLOGY

Outbreaks occur in the winter months (December–March).
Up to 15% of the population may be affected in a year.

. AETIOLOGY AND RISK FACTORS

Influenza is caused by the orthomyxoviruses influenza A, B and C.
- **Influenza A** causes most major influenza outbreaks (pandemics).
- **Influenza B** causes milder, localised outbreaks.
- **Influenza C** causes mild/asymptomatic illness.

Influenza A serotypes can be subdivided on the basis of their surface antigens:
- **Haemagglutinin (H)** facilitates viral entry into host cells.
- **Neuraminidase (N)** facilitates release of new virions from host cells.
- Subtypes are named by combining the H and N numbers e.g. A(H1N1), A(H3N2).
- Influenza has a propensity to undergo mutation and form new viral subtypes:
  - **Antigenic drift:** Minor mutations to the H or N surface antigens. This causes small seasonal epidemics only as partial immunity exists within the population.
  - **Antigenic shift:** Major changes to H or N surface antigens, resulting in the emergence of a new viral subtype. There is little/no population immunity so a major epidemic or pandemic may result.

Respiratory Medicine

MICRO-print

Influenza Pandemics

- **Spanish Flu (1918–1920):** a global pandemic of H1N1.
  - It was the most devastating of the 20th century; responsible for ~50 million deaths.
- **Asian Flu (1957–1958):** a strain of H2N2 avian flu originating in China with a worldwide death toll of 1–4 million.
- **Hong Kong Flu (1968–1969):** a strain of H3N2, caused by antigenic shift from a pre-existing H2N2 strain.
  - It was responsible for ~1 million deaths.
- **Swine Flu (2009–2010):** originated in Mexico.
  - It is thought to be due to a strain of H1N1 caused by a mutation of four existing H1N1 strains.
  - WHO reported that over 18209 deaths were caused by the virus as of 20 June 2010.

- **Transmission:**
  - Respiratory droplet spread or through direct contact with infectious material.
- **Risk factors**
  - Pre-existing respiratory disease (e.g. asthma, cystic fibrosis).
  - Pre-existing cardiac/chronic disease.
  - Older age.
  - Close contact between individuals e.g. residential homes.

4. CLINICAL FEATURES

- **Incubation period:** 1–3 days.
- **Acute illness:**
  - **Symptoms:**
    - Fever
    - Myalgia
    - Headache
    - Sore throat
    - Dry cough.
  - **Signs:**
    - Pyrexia
    - Mild cervical lymphadenopathy.

- **Post-viral syndrome:**
    - Prolonged period of debility or depression.
    - May last for weeks to months.

5. INVESTIGATIONS

- Usually a clinical diagnosis.
- Investigations are used for community surveillance and include:
    - Immunofluorescence of nasopharyngeal swab/aspirate.
    - Viral culture of nasopharyngeal swab/aspirate.
    - Acute and convalescent sera, 1–2 weeks apart.
    - PCR.
- PCR-based tests are the most commonly used diagnostic test, and point-of-care testing (POCT) in emergency departments is becoming commonplace allowing rapid diagnosis/exclusion.
- For patients presenting to hospital, a chest X-ray is usually performed to evaluate for pneumonitis and to exclude other causes of symptoms e.g. pneumonia.

6. DIFFERENTIAL DIAGNOSIS

- **Upper respiratory tract infection**
- **Lower respiratory tract infection**
- Pneumonia
- Infectious mononucleosis
- Cytomegalovirus
- HIV seroconversion
- Malaria (in returning travellers).

7. MANAGEMENT

- **Supportive care:**
    - Bed rest
    - Increase fluid intake
    - Analgesics (e.g. paracetamol)
    - Antipyretics (e.g. paracetamol).
- **Antivirals:** Neuraminidase inhibitors (e.g. oseltamivir, zanamivir) are recommended for "at risk" individuals (see below).
- **Infection control measures:**
    - Handwashing.
    - Appropriate use of personal protective equipment (PPE).
    - Segregation of pandemic influenza cases away from patients with other medical problems.
    - Barrier nursing.
- **Prevention:** Vaccination (see below).

Respiratory Medicine

> ## MICRO-facts
>
> Influenza vaccines are administered annually to those considered at risk:
>
> - Patients aged >65.
> - Pregnant women.
> - Immunocompromised patients.
> - Those in long-stay residential facilities.
> - Carers.
> - Patients with chronic respiratory, cardiac, renal, liver or neurological disease; or those with diabetes mellitus.
>
> Each year, a new vaccine is produced based on recommendations from the WHO regarding the strains of influenza which should be protected against. The UK uses a trivalent vaccine against two influenza A strains and one influenza B strain. Influenza vaccines are inactive and therefore safe for use in immunocompromised individuals.

8. COMPLICATIONS

- **Respiratory complications:**
  - **Secondary bacterial pneumonia** (usually *Streptococcus pneumoniae*)
  - Primary viral pneumonia
  - Asthma/COPD exacerbations.
- **Non-respiratory complications:**
  - **General:** toxic shock syndrome associated with *Staphylococcus aureus*.
  - **Cardiac:** myocarditis, heart failure.
  - **Neurological:** encephalitis, transverse myelitis, Guillain-Barré syndrome.
  - **Musculoskeletal:** myositis.

9. PROGNOSIS

- Recovery usually within 1–2 weeks.
- Mortality highest in infants, elderly and those with pre-existing co-morbidities.
- Worldwide, over 20,000 deaths a year are attributed to seasonal influenza.

> ### MICRO-case
> You are an SHO working in A&E when you are asked to see an acutely unwell 78-year-old man, who suffers with COPD. He has had an acute exacerbation of his condition, experiencing increased breathlessness associated with symptoms of sore throat, headache, back and thigh pain, and a persistent dry cough. He tells you *continued...*

continued...   he feels feverish and has been "shaking". The symptoms have been present for ~4 days. Through careful history-taking you discover that he did not attend the appointment for his annual influenza vaccination. His 10-year-old grandson was recently off school with symptoms of cough, headache and muscle pains, although he recovered within a week. Vital signs reveal a pulse of 80, RR of 26, temperature of $38.2°C$, BP of $124/86$ and O_2 Sats of 84%.

You request a chest X-ray, which reveals no consolidation. However, based on your initial assessment, you recommend admission and begin treatment with oxygen therapy, intravenous fluids and simple analgesia. You suspect a diagnosis of influenza, and although his symptoms have been present for greater than 48 hours, antiviral therapy with Tamiflu (oseltamivir) is commenced due to the continuing symptoms and high risk of complications. He is nursed in a side room and staff are reminded to wear aprons and gloves and follow normal handwashing procedure to prevent the spread of influenza to the other patients on the respiratory ward. A PCR throat swab later confirms the diagnosis.

Key Points
- Influenza is usually an uncomplicated self-limiting infection in the young fit patient but is a major cause of morbidity and mortality in the elderly or those with pre-existing chronic diseases. Flu vaccination is an effective means of preventing infection and is offered to all those "at risk" of influenza.
- Antivirals (e.g. Tamiflu) may be prescribed in individuals at high risk of complications. (see above). Ideally, antiviral treatment should be commenced within 48 hours of symptom onset.

2.3 ACUTE BRONCHITIS

1. DEFINITION

- Inflammation of the large airways (bronchi).

2. EPIDEMIOLOGY

- Affecting $44/1000$ adults every year.
- Increased prevalence in the autumn and winter months.

3. AETIOLOGY AND RISK FACTORS

- **Viral bronchitis:** viral infections (e.g. coronavirus, rhinovirus) are the commonest causes of bronchitis in previously healthy individuals.
- **Bacterial bronchitis:** secondary bacterial infection may occur following viral infection and is associated with pre-existing respiratory disease (e.g. COPD), and smoking.

4. PATHOPHYSIOLOGY

- Inflammation of the bronchi may occur in response to a viral or bacterial infective trigger, or an environmental irritant.
- This is associated with increased mucus production within the bronchi.
  - This is responsible for the characteristic productive cough.

5. CLINICAL FEATURES

- **Symptoms:**
  - **Cough:** initially unproductive, later productive of yellow/green sputum.
  - Discomfort behind sternum.
  - Chest tightness.
  - Wheeze.
  - Shortness of breath.
- **Signs:**
  - **On auscultation:** wheeze.

6. INVESTIGATIONS

- **Sputum:** culture and microscopy.
- **Chest X-ray:** consider to exclude pneumonia.

7. DIFFERENTIAL DIAGNOSIS

- Influenza
- Pharyngitis
- Sinusitis.

8. MANAGEMENT

- Often resolves with rest and increased fluid intake.
- **Symptomatic treatment:** analgesia, antipyretics.
- **Antibiotics** such as amoxicillin may be prescribed in those with increased risk of developing subsequent pneumonia.

9. COMPLICATIONS

- **Pneumonia** may occur if the infection spreads distally through the airways.

10. PROGNOSIS

- In healthy individuals, resolution within 4–8 days.
- Risk of complications or a longer duration of illness is increased in those with pre-existing lung disease and in smokers.

Respiratory Medicine

2.4 COMMUNITY-ACQUIRED PNEUMONIA (CAP)

1. DEFINITION

- Pneumonia is a disease that leads to consolidation of the lung parenchyma.
  - It is characterised by acute inflammation in alveoli, as well as the respiratory and terminal bronchioles, with an infiltration of neutrophils.
- The consolidation is either in bronchopulmonary segments (**bronchopneumonia**) or involves an entire lobe (**lobar pneumonia**; see Figures 2.1 and 2.2).
- There are also non-infectious idiopathic pneumonias (such as usual interstitial pneumonia [UIP] and cryptogenic organising pneumonia [COP]), which are considered in Chapter 12.

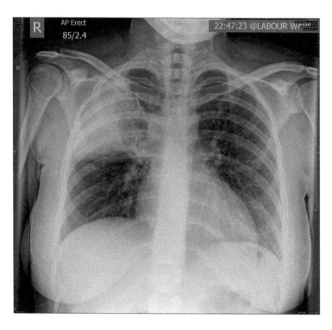

Figure 2.1 Chest X-ray of patient with right-sided upper lobe pneumonia; opacity is seen in the right upper lobe, indicating lobar consolidation.

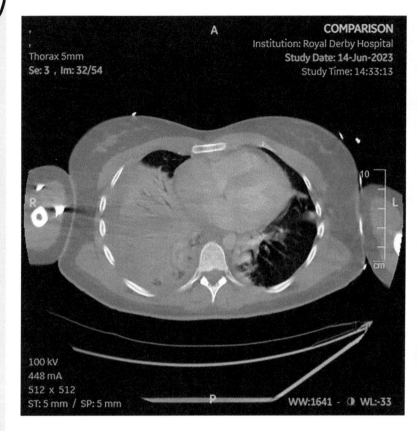

Figure 2.2 CT chest of a patient with right-sided upper lobe pneumonia.

2. EPIDEMIOLOGY

- Community-acquired pneumonia has an incidence of 5–11 per 1,000 in the UK.
- The rate of hospital admission is approximately 1 per 1,000 /year.
- Pneumonia is the fifth leading cause of death in the UK.

3. AETIOLOGY AND RISK FACTORS

- Pneumonia can be caused by a variety of organisms: bacterial, viral, fungal, protozoal.
  - Community-acquired pneumonia is most commonly caused by *S. pneumoniae* (see Table 2.1 for important causative pathogens).
- **Risk factors:**
  - Female (3:1 predominance).
  - Young or elderly (<16 yrs or >65 yrs).
  - Chronic heart or lung disease (e.g. COPD, CF, bronchiectasis).

Table 2.1 Common pathogens causing community-acquired pneumonia.

COMMON PATHOGENS	FEATURES	CASES (%)
Streptococcus pneumoniae	High susceptibility to penicillin.	30–54%
Haemophilus influenzae	Causative pathogen in young children and those with underlying lung disease or immunodeficiency.	6–15%
Mycoplasma pneumonia	Cyclical epidemics in young adults every few years.	18%
Legionella pneumophilia	Found in stagnant humidified water. Sporadic outbreaks. High mortality (30%). Associated with high fever, rigors, myalgia, headache and ataxia.	2–7%
Staphylococcus aureus	Common in IV drug users, alcoholics and those with mitral valve disease. Causes cavitating pneumonia.	2%

- Smoking and environmental pollutants.
- Compromised immune system (e.g. HIV/AIDS, malignancy, splenectomy, diabetes mellitus).
- Alcohol and drug abuse.

MICRO-facts

Atypical pneumonia is caused by less common organisms that are harder to identify through standard microbiological tests (i.e. not *Streptococcus pneumoniae*, *Haemophilus influenza* or *Moraxella catarrhalis*). Examples include:

- *Mycoplasma pneumoniae*
- Legionella pneumophilia
- Chlamydophilia pneumoniae
- Chlamydophilia psittaci.

Atypical organisms are considered more likely to cause an unusual or systemic presentation. An atypical organism is suggested if:

- The pneumonia does not respond to penicillin.
- There is no lobar consolidation.
- There are extra-pulmonary symptoms.
- There is absence of leucocytosis.
- There is moderate or no sputum production.
- There are few physical signs, compared to symptom profile.

Identifying an atypical cause can be important, as it may not respond to standard first-line therapy.

Respiratory Medicine

4. PATHOPHYSIOLOGY

- Majority of serious CAP are **bacterial:**
  - Colonisation of upper airway by pathogen.
  - Translocation of pathogen into lower airway.
  - Infiltration of neutrophils: cytokine release.
  - Inflammation and oedema.
  - Consolidation.
  - Resolution (+/– chronic damage and scarring) or death.

5. CLINICAL FEATURES

- **Symptoms:**
  - Cough, sometimes with haemoptysis.
  - Sputum which is usually discoloured, although cough may be dry.
  - Dyspnoea.
  - Pleuritic chest pain.
  - Referred abdominal pain.
  - Vomiting.
  - Confusion (cause of acute confusional state in elderly).
  - Myalgia + arthralgia.
  - Malaise.
- **Signs:**
  - Fever
  - Tachycardia
  - Tachypnoea
  - Cyanosis
  - Chest signs:
    - ↓ Chest expansion
    - Dullness on percussion
    - ↑ Vocal/tactile fremitus
    - Bronchial breathing
    - Crepitations/crackles
    - Whispering pectoriloquy/bronchophony
    - ↓ Air entry.

6. INVESTIGATIONS

- Full blood count (FBC) (with white cell differential).
- U+Es (performed to assess CURB-65 score; see Table 2.2).
- Chest X-ray.
- Pulse oximetry (arterial blood gas may be required).
- Sputum culture and Gram stain.
- Point-of-care PCR for respiratory viruses (COVID-19/influenza).
- Special tests: urinary legionella and pneumococcal antigen testing.
- HIV testing: pneumonia often initial presentation.

. DIFFERENTIAL DIAGNOSIS

» Tuberculosis.
» Acute bronchitis.
» Lung malignancy.
  Aspiration of upper airway secretions, vomitus, or foreign body.
  Bronchiectasis.

. MANAGEMENT

» Decision on whether to admit based on clinical judgment and by using the
  CURB-65 score (see Table 2.2). Note that this score is only validated for
  community-acquired pneumonia, not for other respiratory infections. It is a
  predictor of mortality, with the higher the score, the higher the risk of death.

Table 2.2 **CURB-65 community-acquired pneumonia prognostic score.**

CURB-65 PNEUMONIA TREATMENT SCORE	Points
Confusion	1
Urea ≥7 mmol/L	1
Respiratory rate >30	1
Blood Pressure ≤ 90/60 mmHg	1
≥65 years old	1
Management algorithm	
Manage as an outpatient	0–1
Admit to hospital (short-stay)	2
Admit to hospital + consider level 2 or 3 care setting	3+

Antibiotic therapy: antibiotic therapy generally follows local treatment
guidelines and are often based on CURB-65 score. Typical oral regimes
(NICE and BTS guidance) are:
- Amoxicillin 500 mg TDS + clarithromycin 500 mg BD for 5 days.
- Suspected penicillin resistance: macrolide or doxycycline 100 mg BD
  for 5 days.
- Aspiration pneumonia: co-amoxiclav.

If CURB-65 ≥3:
- Co-amoxiclav 1.2 g IV TDS with IV/oral clarithromycin 500 mg BD.

IV fluid replacement: if patient is hypotensive or dehydrated.
Thromboprophylaxis: if appropriate after risk assessment.
Analgesia: e.g. paracetamol.

Respiratory Medicine

9. COMPLICATIONS

- Respiratory failure.
- Parapneumonic effusion.
- Empyema (see Chapter 2 section 5).
- Lung abscess.
- Bronchiectasis.

10. PROGNOSIS

- Most bacterial pneumonias with appropriate antibiotic treatment will improve within a week.
- X-ray changes should resolve within:
  - 6 weeks in patients <60 yrs.
  - 6 weeks + a week per decade past 60 in patients >60 yrs.
- Mortality is about 1%, but rises to between 5.7 and 14% in the subpopulation that are hospitalised with CAP.
- **Prevention:**
  - Smoking cessation
  - Appropriate antibiotic prescribing
  - Pneumococcal + influenza vaccinations.

MICRO-references

For more detail on the investigation and management of an adult patient with community-acquired pneumonia, including use of the CURB-65 score, the reader should access the British Thoracic Society guidance:

www.brit-thoracic.org.uk/Portals/0/Clinical%20Information/Pneumonia/Guidelines/CAPQuickRefGuide-web.pdf

---

MICRO-case

You are an SHO working in A&E. A young woman brings in her grandfather, Alfred, a 72-year-old pensioner. She says that he has had a cough for the last few days and has been generally unwell. However, she tells you that over the last few hours he seems to have had problems breathing. When you go to see him he is confused and is not orientated to place or person. When you take his vital signs, he has a RR 29, BP 115 / 65, temperature 39°C and a pulse of 82. On examination of the chest you note dullness on percussion at the left base, and on auscultation you hear coarse crackles. When his blood results come back from the lab, his WCC and CRP are raised, but his urea and glucose are normal. A chest X-ray shows consolidation at the left lung base. You calculate that his CURB-65 score is 2 and so decide that he should *continued..*

continued...
be admitted as an inpatient. You start IV fluids and empirical antibiotics and send blood cultures and sputum cultures to the lab. He is kept under close observation for any change in his clinical condition. He deteriorates and his blood pressure drops to 88 / 50 and his RR is now 35, at which point you ask for senior review and a decision is made that he should be transferred to the critical care unit. His CURB-65 score at this point is 4.

Key Points
- Always try to get a collateral history e.g. from family/carer.
- This is especially important if the patient is confused or has reduced levels of consciousness.
- Always calculate a CURB-65 score for a patient with suspected pneumonia: it can be used to guide management decisions.
- Initially, this gentleman had a "moderate severity" score and would need managing as an inpatient.
- However, he deteriorates and now has a "high severity" score (4), so senior review and transfer to ITU is indicated.
- CURB-65 is also useful as a prognostic index (e.g. a score of 4 has approximately a 40% risk of mortality).
- Always frequently re-assess acutely ill patients.
- Management decisions may need to be adjusted in line with the patient's clinical condition.
- Always obtain a baseline CRP and WCC, as repeat measurements will then allow assessment of the patient's response to treatment.
- Treatment failure or atypical changes on chest X-ray (e.g. cavitation) may indicate an atypical organism.
- Start empirical antibiotic therapy as soon as possible.
- Always try to send blood and sputum cultures for MC&S.
- This allows tailoring of future antibiotic therapy.
- If possible, take samples before initiation of empirical antibiotic therapy.

2.5 HOSPITAL-ACQUIRED PNEUMONIA (HAP)

. DEFINITION

Hospital-acquired (nosocomial) pneumonia (HAP) refers to new consolidation.
- Onset is at least 48 hours after admission to hospital or within 6 weeks of discharge.
- Higher morbidity and mortality than CAP.

. EPIDEMIOLOGY

HAP occurs in 5–15 patients per 1,000 hospital admissions.
In the important subgroup of patients on mechanical ventilation this rises to 10 − 25 episodes per 1,000 ventilator days.

3. AETIOLOGY AND RISK FACTORS

- Gram-negatives are the predominant organisms in hospital-acquired pneumonia:
    - *Escherichia coli.*
    - *Klebsiella pneumonia.*
    - *Pseudomonas aeruginosa.*
- Antibiotic-resistant strains are more prevalent in the hospital setting.
    - Pneumonias are associated with a higher rate of treatment failure.
- **Aetiology:** Likely infective organisms are dependent on the period of onset (relative to the patients admission) of the illness (atypical organisms are described in the MICRO-Facts box below):
    - **Early onset (<4 days):** *S. pneumoniae, Haemophilus influenzae, Moraxella catarrhalis.*
    - **Late onset (>4 days):** gram-negative organisms, *S. aureus, Legionella pneumophilia.*
    - It is also important to consider hospital-acquired viral infection such as COVID-19 or influenza, especially during pandemics.
- **Risk factors:** are the same as those for CAP but also include:
    - Use of invasive devices: intubation, nasogastric tube, nasotracheal tube.
    - Prior antibiotic use.
    - Hyperglycaemia.
    - Obesity.
    - Decreased consciousness.
    - Suppressed cough reflex (e.g. post-surgery and use of sedatives, narcotics or neuromuscular blockade).

4. PATHOPHYSIOLOGY

- Aspiration from the digestive tract is the most common route of infection in hospital-acquired pneumonia.
- Due to this, there are high rates of mixed organism infections.
- Local trauma and inflammation from mechanical ventilation aid colonisation.

5. CLINICAL FEATURES

- Presentation is usually the same as CAP and should always be considered when a patient in hospital shows new respiratory symptoms or a non-specific deterioration in their condition.

6. INVESTIGATIONS

- Same as for a patient with CAP.
- Bronchoscopy + broncho-alveolar lavage (BAL) if there is diagnostic uncertainty.

- Consider chest CT: aids in the diagnosis of complications such as empyema + lung abscess.

7. DIFFERENTIAL DIAGNOSIS

- Same differential diagnosis to CAP, but also consider:
    - Pulmonary embolus.
    - Pneumothorax.
    - Pulmonary oedema.
    - Acute respiratory distress syndrome (ARDS).
    - Congestive heart failure.

8. MANAGEMENT

- **IV antibiotics:** typical regimes in HAP (taken from NICE guidelines, please check local guidelines) are:
    - Piperacillin/tazobactam 4.5 g IV TDS.
    - If penicillin allergic: meropenem 2 g IV TDS (discuss with micro-biology; meropenem is not always appropriate if penicillin causes anaphylaxis).
    - Early antibiotic therapy improves outcomes, so empirical coverage should be started and then streamlined once sensitivities are known.
    - Antibiotic treatment should be guided by culture and sensitivity.
- **Analgesia** (use WHO analgesia ladder as a guide for effective analgesia).
- **Thromboprophylaxis.**
- **IV fluid replacement.**
- **Chest physiotherapy.**
- **Prevention:**
    - Handwashing + proper infection control strategies.
    - Early identification and mitigation of swallowing problems (common in elderly or patients with dementia).
    - Removal of invasive devices as soon as possible.
    - Nursing in semi-upright position.
    - Limited use of sedatives.
    - Early weaning from ventilation.

9. COMPLICATIONS

- Hospital-acquired pneumonia has the same complications as CAP.

10. PROGNOSIS

- Pneumonia treated in hospital has a mortality rate of $6-12\%$ (majority of which are CAP).
- HAP has a mortality rate of approximately 30%.
- Mortality approximately 50% for pneumonia requiring treatment in ITU.

Respiratory Medicine

2.6 EMPYEMA (PYOTHORAX)

1. DEFINITION

- Accumulation of pus or culture-positive fluid within pleural space, usually complicating bacterial pneumonia.
- Non-purulent culture negative fluid with pH < 7.2 (complicated parapneumonic fluid) should be managed as empyema.

2. EPIDEMIOLOGY

- Small amounts of non-purulent fluid in the pleural space (parapneumonic effusion) is commonly found in patients with pneumonia, especially if CT scan or thoracic USS is undertaken for any reason.
- 5% of patients with pneumonia progress to empyema.
- 2:1 male-female ratio.

3. AETIOLOGY AND RISK FACTORS

- 70% are secondary to pneumonia.
- Other causes: iatrogenic or trauma, oesophageal tear/rupture (Boerhaave's syndrome)
- Infective organisms depend on the aetiology:
  - **Community acquired:** *Streptococcus milleri, Streptococcus pneumoniae.*
  - **Hospital acquired:** *Staphylococci* (particularly MRSA).
- **Risk factors:**
  - Aspiration
  - Immunocompromise
  - Alcohol and drug abuse
  - Thoracic surgery
  - Chest drain insertion
  - Thoracocentesis.

4. PATHOPHYSIOLOGY

- The bacteria spread to the pleural cavity through the lymphatic system, most often from a primary site within the lung.
- An empyema can progress from an initially sterile pleural effusion – it classically forms in three stages (see Figure 2.3).

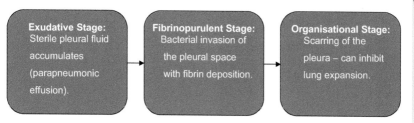

Figure 2.3 Pathophysiology of empyema.

5. CLINICAL FEATURES

- Classical presentation: persistent swinging fever, leucocytosis and failure to improve following 4–5 days of antibiotic therapy for pneumonia.
- **Symptoms:**
    - Pleuritic chest pain
    - Dyspnoea
    - Cough
    - Malaise
    - Night sweats
    - Anorexia.
- **Signs:**
    - Swinging fever
    - Rigors
    - Chest signs:
        - ↓ Chest expansion.
        - ↓ Tactile fremitus.
        - Tracheal deviation towards empyema – rare.
        - Stony dullness on percussion.
        - Pleural rub.
        - ↓ Vocal resonance.
        - ↓ Breath sounds.

Respiratory Medicine

6. INVESTIGATIONS

- FBC + white cell differential.
- CRP.
- Serum LDH (to compare to pleural fluid).
- Chest X-ray (see Figure 2.4).
- CT (see Figure 2.5).
- Ultrasound-guided thoracocentesis (needle aspiration) is a key investigation in determining the cause and guiding treatment:
  - Gram stain + culture
  - Fluid protein, glucose + LDH
  - Cytology (see Chapter 1).

7. DIFFERENTIAL DIAGNOSIS

- Pneumonia (atypical)
- Uncomplicated para-pneumonic effusion
- Lung abscess
- Malignant effusion
- Oesophageal rupture.

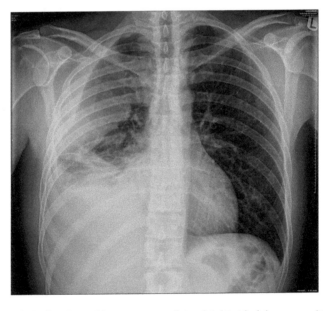

Figure 2.4 CXR of patient with empyema; unilateral right-sided dense opacity in lower section of right lung.

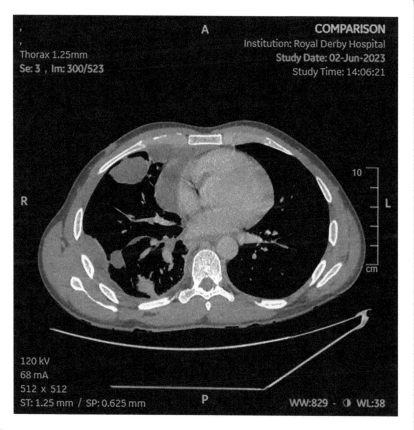

Figure 2.5 Chest CT of patient with empyema in the pleural space around the right lung.

8. MANAGEMENT

- Empirical IV antibiotic coverage in line with local guidelines, typically:
  - Community acquired: co-amoxiclav 1.2 g IV TDS, 625 mg PO TDS.
  - Hospital acquired: piperacillin/tazobactam (Tazocin) 4.5 g TDS.
- Further antibiotic coverage should be guided by culture and sensitivity, usually including anaerobic cover. It may be necessary to continue antibiotics for several weeks.
- Analgesia + antipyretics.
- Chest-drain insertion may be needed depending on the microbiological, biochemical and physical properties of the effusion. Purulent fluid, low pH, larger effusions are more likely to need a drain.

Respiratory Medicine

- Video-assisted thoracoscopic surgery (VATS) for decortication and debridement if previous measures fail (after 5–7 days of treatment), or if the fluid is heavily loculated predicting failure of tube drainage.
- Intrapleural fibrinolytics (urokinase or streptokinase) in limited selected cases where surgery is not appropriate.

9. COMPLICATIONS

- Respiratory failure.
- Unilateral pulmonary oedema: secondary to fluid drainage (rare).
- Uncontrolled infection and sepsis.
- Chronic trapped lung due to persistent fluid and/or pleural thickening.

10. PROGNOSIS

- Majority of patients respond fully to antibiotics and tube drainage.
- Up to 30% of patients require surgery.
- 15–20% mortality rate following empyema.

2.7 COVID-19

1. DEFINITION

- COVID-19 is a viral respiratory tract infection, caused by the novel SARS-CoV-2 virus.
    - First identified in late 2019 in the Hubei province of China.
    - Cause of a global pandemic and now an endemic illness.
- Most commonly it causes mild upper respiratory tract illness.
- In a proportion of cases it can progress to pneumonia or multi-system disease.

2. EPIDEMIOLOGY

- A worldwide pandemic was declared in March 2020 shortly after identification of the virus.
- As of May 2023, over 765 million confirmed cases and nearly 7 million deaths were reported globally (https://covid19.who.int).
- In the UK there were 21 million cases and 226,000 deaths (https://coronavirus.data.gov.uk).
- Following the introduction of a worldwide vaccination programme, incidence has fallen and severe disease is much less common.

3. AETIOLOGY AND RISK FACTORS

- A coronavirus spread by droplet, airborne and fomite transmission.
- Risk factors (for poor outcome):
    - Age
    - Male sex

- Obesity
- Pregnancy
- Chronic disease
- Immunosuppression/immunodeficiency.

4. CLINICAL FEATURES

Incubation period:
- 5–14 days

Acute illness:
- **Symptoms:**
- Due to antigenic drift there are multiple variants with variable symptomatology:
  - Majority: asymptomatic/mild coryza
  - Fever
  - Cough
  - Tiredness
  - Loss of sense of taste and smell
  - Headache
  - Muscle aches
  - Chest pain
  - Shortness of breath
- **Signs:**
  - Majority: None/mild coryza
  - Respiratory distress
  - Fever
  - Tachycardia
  - Tachypnoea
  - Cyanosis.
    - Chest signs:
    - ↓ Chest expansion
    - Dullness on percussion
    - ↑ Vocal/tactile fremitus
    - Bronchial breathing
    - Crepitations/crackles
    - Whispering pectoriloquy/bronchophony
    - ↓ Air entry.

5. INVESTIGATIONS

Rapid antigen/lateral flow tests
- Considerably less sensitive than RT-PCR.
- Require a nasopharyngeal or oropharyngeal swab.
- Rapid and inexpensive to perform.

Respiratory Medicine

- Able to detect the majority of infectious cases (i.e. individuals with a high viral load).
- A negative test, particularly in a symptomatic patient, does not exclude COVID-19, and RT-PCR should be performed if clinical suspicion remains.
- Available in the community as well as secondary care settings.
- RT-PCR
  - Require a nasopharyngeal or oropharyngeal swab in early stage disease.
  - Consider a sputum sample, endotracheal swab or bronchoalveaolar lavage (BAL) in late stage or severe disease.
  - A positive test confirms a diagnosis of COVID-19.
- Blood tests
  - Evaluation is similar to patient with other respiratory infections and depending on severity will usually include FBC, U&E, LFT, CRP, clotting.
  - ABG if suspected respiratory failure.
  - Blood culture/sputum/culture/urinary antigens to look for alternative c secondary infection.
  - Procalcitonin:
    - Elevation of procalcitonin is associated with more severe disease and higher mortality. It is also elevated by secondary bacterial infection.
- Imaging
  - CXR: Indicated if SpO2 < 94% on air, NEWS2 ≥ 3 or if clinical suspi cion of pneumonia.
    - May show ground glass opacification or consolidation.
    - Typically bilateral, peripheral and basal distribution.
  - CT
- Consider for seriously unwell patients with normal CXR.

6. DIFFERENTIAL DIAGNOSIS

- Influenza.
- Bacterial pneumonia.
  - Community acquired.
  - Hospital acquired.
  - Aspiration.
  - Atypical organisms including *Pneumocystis jirovecii*.
- Common cold and other coryzal illness.
- Other bacterial or viral respiratory infections.

. MANAGEMENT

- **Community management**
  - Self-isolation.
  - Antipyretics.
  - **Specific treatment for patients at highest risk of progression (see MICRO-Facts, below):**
    - **Antivirals:** nirmatrelvir and ritonavir (Paxlovid), remdesivir (Veklury), molnupiravir (Lagevrio).
    - **Neutralising monoclonal antibodies:** sotrovimab (Xevudy).
    - Used if antivirals are contraindicated.
- **Indications for admission**
  - Hypoxia
  - Severely unwell patient.

MICRO-facts

Patient groups considered "at highest risk of progression":

- Chromosomal disorders affecting the immune system, including Down's syndrome.
- Certain types of cancer or have received treatment for certain types of cancer.
- Sickle cell disease.
- Chronic kidney disease (CKD) stage 4 or 5.
- Severe liver disease.
- Had an organ transplant.
- Autoimmune or inflammatory conditions (such as rheumatoid arthritis or inflammatory bowel disease).
- Inherited or acquired conditions affecting their immune system.
- Rare neurological conditions: multiple sclerosis, motor neurone disease, Huntington's disease or myasthenia gravis.

Secondary care management
Supportive
- Oxygen therapy
- Antipyretics
- VTE prophylaxis.

Corticosteroids: The RECOVERY trial (www.nejm.org/doi/10.1056/NEJMoa2021436) showed that dexamethasone (6 mg daily) reduces 28-day mortality.

Respiratory Medicine

- Recommended for all patients where pneumonitis is causing a need for supplemental oxygen to maintain target saturations.
- Continue for up to 10 days, stopping when oxygen requirement resolves.
- Commonly cause rises in blood sugars which should be monitored and treated according to local guidelines.
- Prednisolone and hydrocortisone can be used if dexamethasone contraindicated.
- **Interleukin-6 (IL-6) inhibitors:** tocilizumab, sarilizumab.
  - Recommended for patients with more severe disease, where there is no evidence of another bacterial or viral infection that may be worsened by an IL-6 inhibitor.
  - Usually given if requiring additional respiratory support beyond low flow rates of oxygen (i.e. HFNC, CPAP, assisted ventilation).
  - Also given in less severe cases where CRP > 75 mg/L.
- **Baricitinib:** A Janus kinase (JAK) inhibitor.
  - If needing supplemental oxygen.
  - Requiring, or have completed, a course of corticosteroids.
  - No evidence of another bacterial or viral infection that might be worsened by baricitinib.
- If there is deterioration despite an IL-6 inhibitor or baricitinib, it may be appropriate to add a drug from the other class.
- **Antibiotics**
  - Only use if there is evidence/suspicion of superadded bacterial infection.
- **Prone positioning**
  - Consider awake proning for patients who are not intubated and have higher oxygen needs.
  - Reduces ventilation/perfusion mismatch, hypoxaemia and shunting.
- **Continuous positive airway pressure (CPAP)**
  - Recommended in patients not responding to supplemental oxygen with $FiO2 > 0.4$ (40%).
  - For patients who would be considered for invasive mechanical ventilation but do not have an immediate need for it; or patients for whom there is an agreement that respiratory support should not be escalated to invasive medical ventilation.
- **High-flow nasal oxygen (HFNO)**
  - Should not be routinely offered as the main form of respiratory support in patients that would be suitable for invasive mechanical ventilation or CPAP.
- **Invasive mechanical ventilation**
  - Decisions to escalate to invasive mechanical ventilation (and indeed all forms of respiratory support) should be based on the person's likelihood of recovery.

- **Prevention**
  - **Infection control measures:**
    - Handwashing.
    - Appropriate use of personal protective equipment (PPE).
    - Segregation of positive cases away from patients with other medical problems.
    - Barrier nursing.
  - **Vaccination:** See MICRO-facts

MICRO-facts

The UK COVID-19 vaccination program began in December 2020, starting with patients most vulnerable to severe illness from COVID-19. For most vaccines, the course consists of an initial vaccination followed by a booster at 12 weeks. Further booster doses are offered dependent on clinical risk.

The COVID-19 vaccines currently approved and in use in the UK are:

- mRNA vaccines: Moderna (Spikevax) and Pfizer/BioNTech (Comirnaty).
- Novavax (Nuvaxovid): protein subunit vaccine.
- Other vaccines – e.g. the adenovirus vector vaccines made by AstraZeneca and Janssen – are approved but not currently available.

COMPLICATIONS

Respiratory complications:
- Acute respiratory distress syndrome (ARDS)
- Secondary bacterial pneumonia:
  - Rare
  - Increased risk in the immunocompromised

Non-respiratory complications:
- Sepsis
- Multiorgan failure
- Acute kidney injury
- Acute liver injury
- Venous thromboembolism
- **Cardiovascular:** heart failure, acute coronary syndrome, arrhythmia
- **Neurological:** including CVA, seizures, ataxia, encephalopathy, cerebral venous sinus thrombosis, peripheral neuropathy, myopathy.

Respiratory Medicine

- **Post–COVID-19 syndrome ("long Covid")**
  - Definitions vary:
    - **WHO:** "a condition that occurs in people with a history of probable or confirmed SARS-CoV-2 infection, usually occurring 3 months from the onset of symptoms and lasting for at least 2 months, that cannot be explained by an alternative diagnosis".
    - **NICE:** "signs and symptoms that develop during or after an infection consistent with COVID-19, continue for more than 12 weeks, and are not explained by an alternative diagnosis".

9. PROGNOSIS

- Risk of death in patients <65 years old and without comorbidities is low.
- Mortality rates have fallen since the beginning of the pandemic.
  - Factors include better hospital processes for managing COVID-19 positive patients, adherence to evidence-based guidelines, vaccination uptake and emergence of less virulent strains of the virus.
- The main cause of death from COVID-19 is ARDS.
  - The overall mortality rate from Covid-related ARDS is 39%.

MICRO-references
COVID-19 rapid guideline: Managing COVID-19 – The National Institute for Health and Care Excellence. Available at: www.nice.org.uk/guidance/ng191/resources/covid19-rapid-guideline- managing-covid19-pdf-51035553326

Asthma

1. DEFINITION

- Asthma is a chronic inflammatory disorder affecting large and small airways associated with:
  - Airway hyper-responsiveness
  - Variable airflow obstruction.

2. EPIDEMIOLOGY

- Asthma affects around 1 in 11 children and 1 in 12 adults in the UK.
- Asthma prevalence is on the increase worldwide.
- Traditionally the peak age of diagnosis is 5–15 years old, with a second peak in the sixth decade of life; however, some adults may have persistent subclinical symptoms which manifest more prominently in middle-age.

3. AETIOLOGY AND RISK FACTORS

- Atopy: a triad of asthma, eczema and food allergies can occur.
- Genetic predisposition.
- Exposure to smoking (including passive smoking).
- Low income.
- Occupation.

4. PATHOPHYSIOLOGY

- The clinical features in asthma are related to two main pathological processes:
  - Airway hyper-responsiveness and bronchospasm
  - Chronic inflammation and remodelling.
- **Airway hyper-responsiveness and bronchospasm:**
  - It is suggested that IgE stimulation is a cause of mast cell degranulation.
  - Mast cell degranulation appears to have a close relationship with bronchial smooth muscle as this event alters contractility.
  - This relationship is complex and not consistent and is only one feature of the pathway to explain airway hyper-responsiveness.

DOI: 10.1201/9781315113937-4

- **Chronic inflammation and remodelling:**
    - Oedema.
    - Cellular infiltration: eosinophils, mast cells, lymphocytes, neutrophils.
    - Disruption of the epithelial lining.
    - Increased smooth muscle.
    - Fibrosis in the subepithelial layer.
    - Mucous gland hypertrophy.

MICRO-print
Phenotyping

The population of patients with asthma has been subdivided based on:

- Demographic status
- Lung function
- Atopic status
- Airway inflammation profile.

This is relevant in the severe asthma population on deciding treatment regimens when British Thoracic Society (BTS) 1–4 (see below) is not effective.

Recognised phenotypes are:

- Early onset and atopic.
- Non-eosinophilic inflammation.
- Late onset disease with eosinophilic inflammation but non-atopic status.

---

5. CLINICAL FEATURES

- The clinical features (see also Table 3.1) are used to classify patients as:
    - **High probability** – diagnosis of asthma likely.
    - **Intermediate probability** – diagnosis uncertain.
    - **Low probability** – diagnosis other than asthma likely.
- The probability of asthma informs subsequent management (see below).
- **Symptoms**
    - Cough
    - Wheeze
    - Shortness of breath
    - Chest tightness.
- **Signs**
    - May be none.
    - **On auscultation:** Expiratory wheeze, prolonged expiratory phase.
    - Chest hyperinflation in long-term poorly controlled asthma.
    - Silent chest – severe life-threatening asthma (see below).

Table 3.1 **Clinical features that increase or decrease the probability of asthma.**

FACTORS THAT INCREASE THE PROBABILITY OF ASTHMA	FACTORS THAT DECREASE THE PROBABILITY OF ASTHMA
• >1 of wheeze, cough, difficulty breathing, chest tightness • Especially if worse at night/early morning; occur in response to exercise/other triggers; occur after taking aspirin or beta blockers • Personal or family history of atopic disorders • Widespread wheeze on auscultation • Otherwise unexplained low FEV_1 or peak flow • Otherwise unexplained eosinophilia	• Prominent dizziness, light-headedness or peripheral tingling • Chronic productive cough in absence of wheeze or breathlessness • Repeatedly normal chest examination when symptomatic • Voice disturbance • Symptoms with colds only • Significant smoking history (>20 pack-years) • Cardiac disease • Normal peak flow/spirometry when symptomatic

- **Important points for history taking**
  - Are the symptoms the same all the time, or do they vary throughout the week/day?
  - Is worsening of symptoms associated with any particular triggers (e.g. pets, pollen, cold air, exercise, occupational exposure)?
  - Are there any nocturnal symptoms?
  - Is there a past medical history of eczema, hay fever or allergy?
  - Is there a family history of asthma?
  - Has the patient tried any bronchodilators and, if so, what effect did these have?
  - Is there a history of smoking?
  - Are there any pets?
  - Are symptoms better away from work i.e. is there occupational asthma? (For more information on occupational asthma, see Chapter 15: Occupational lung disease.)

MICRO-references
British Thoracic Society (BTS) Guideline for Asthma (updated 2019), available at:
www.brit-thoracic.org.uk/quality-improvement/guidelines/asthma/

Respiratory Medicine

6. INVESTIGATIONS

- In adults, lung function tests are performed as part of the routine clinical assessment and patients are stratified as below (see Table 3.2).

Table 3.2 **Management of asthma based on probability and spirometry findings.**

HIGH PROBABILITY OF ASTHMA	INTERMEDIATE PROBABILITY OF ASTHMA	LOW PROBABILITY OF ASTHMA
• Perform a trial of asthma treatment • If responding, continue treatment • If not responding, assess compliance and inhaler technique. Consider further investigation	• Tests for airway obstruction e.g. spirometry, peak flow measurement, challenge tests • Other additional tests include measurement of blood eosinophils, total IgE, IgE to aeroallergens, skin prick tests, exhaled nitric oxide	• Refer as appropriate • Investigate/treat other condition • Assess response and perform further investigation/refer if poor response

- **Spirometry**
  - FEV_1/FVC may show obstructive ratio (<0.7) but may be normal as airflow obstruction is variable.
  - Demonstrable reversibility: increase of > 200 mL (or 15%) in FEV_1 after administration of inhaled β_2-agonists.
- **Flow-Volume Loop**
  - This will demonstrate lower (smaller) airways obstruction:
    - This is characterised by a decrease in flow at lower lung volumes.
- **Airway hyper-responsiveness testing:**
  - Methacholine, histamine and mannitol induce bronchospasm in normal individuals in sufficient amounts.
  - Bronchial hyper-responsiveness is measured as PC_{20}: the minimum dose of the agent which provokes a 20% decrease in FEV_1.
  - PC_{20} will be lower in patients with asthma compared to healthy individuals.
- **Peak expiratory flow rate (PEFR):**
  - Useful in assessing variability and later response to treatment.
    - > 20% diurnal variability on >3 days in the week is highly suggestive.
  - Patients can perform their own PEFR at home and record the results.
  - Sensitivity is only 20%.

- **Establishing specific allergens:**
  - **Skin prick tests:**
    - A small amount of the test substance is introduced to the superficial layers of the epidermis.
    - A wheal >3 mm larger than the control suggests a positive result.
- **Blood tests:**
  - **IgE:** A higher total IgE level is associated with atopic disease.
    - Specific IgE to allergens such as tree and grass pollens, house dust mite and pets can be performed.
    - This can aid management with allergen avoidance.
  - **Eosinophils:** Increased eosinophils are seen in acute exacerbations and poorly controlled disease.
    - Blood eosinophils $> 0.3 x 10^3 cells / \mu L$.
    - Also, consider eosinophilic granulomatosis and polyangiitis (known as Churg-Strauss disease).
- **Fractional exhaled nitric oxide (FeNO):** Non-invasive method which may act as possible surrogate marker for eosinophilic airway inflammation which may influence corticosteroid use.
- **Induced sputum:** Available in a limited number of centres in UK. Presence of sputum eosinophils (>3%) suggests risk of exacerbation and need for increased corticosteroid treatment.

7. DIFFERENTIAL DIAGNOSIS

- **In adults:**
  - Chronic obstructive pulmonary disease (COPD).
  - Tumour or other cause of large airways obstruction.
  - Pulmonary oedema (congestive heart failure – "cardiac asthma").
  - Churg-Strauss disease:
    - Vasculitic process that can mimic severe asthma (see Chapter 11. Interstitial Lung Disease and Vasculitis).
      - ○ Bronchiectasis
      - ○ Interstitial lung disease
      - ○ Post-nasal drip
      - ○ Vocal cord dysfunction
      - ○ Gastro-oesophageal reflux disease
      - ○ Carcinoid syndrome.

8. MANAGEMENT OF CHRONIC ASTHMA

- **Goals of treatment:**
  - The British Thoracic Society (BTS) states that the goal of treatment is control of the disease, defined as:
    - No daytime symptoms.

- No night time awakening due to asthma symptoms.
- No need for rescue medication.
- No exacerbations.
- No limitations on activity.
- Normal lung function (FEV$_1$ or PEFR > 80% predicted/best).

MICRO-facts

The Royal College of Physicians 3 Questions Approach to monitoring asthma:

- In the last month/week, have you had difficulty sleeping because of your asthma?
- Have you had your usual asthma symptoms during the day?
- Has your asthma interfered with your usual daily activities?

One positive = medium morbidity; two/three positive = high morbidity

---

- Minimal medication side effects.
- Different clinical questionnaires are available e.g. asthma control test, RCP 3 Questions Approach to assess impact of disease and control (see MICRO-Facts box).
- **Inhaled Therapy:** there are a lot of different inhalers with different medications, combinations of medications, and delivery systems. Input from a specialist asthma nurse can be critical in choosing the right device (metered dose inhaler vs. dry powder) and checking for adequate inhaler technique. They are generally prescribed according to the BTS Stepwise approach (see Figure 3.2).

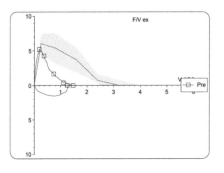 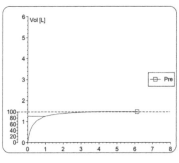

Figure 3.1 Flow volume loop and spirometry: on the left, the flow volume loop shows a reduced lung capacity; on the right, the spirometry shows a reduced FEV$_1$. This is demonstrating a restrictive picture typical of asthma.

- **Short-acting β₂ agonists (SABA):** salbutamol, terbutaline.
  - Take effect quickly (~15 minutes) and last 4–6 hours.
  - Side effects may include tremor, palpitations and muscle cramps.
  - Short-acting anticholinergic/antimuscarinic bronchodilators are rarely used now as long-acting compounds are more effective (see below).
- **Long-acting β₂ agonists (LABA):** salmeterol, formoterol.
  - Similar side effect profile to SABA.
  - Formoterol has more rapid onset than salmeterol.
  - Increased risk of mortality with monotherapy use so expected to be given in combination with an inhaled steroid (can be combined in a single inhaler).
- **Long-acting anticholinergic/anti-muscarinic (LAMA):** tiotropium bromide.
  - Can be considered as add-on therapy in patients poorly controlled on ICS/LABA.
  - Commonly causes dry mouth.
  - Caution in severe renal impairment.
- **Inhaled corticosteroids (ICS):** beclamethasone diproprionate (BDP), budesonide, fluticasone, mometasone.
  - The most effective preventative therapy.
  - Reduces symptoms, exacerbations and improves lung function with an impact on airway inflammation.
  - Have a low threshold for starting in any symptomatic patient but strongly consider in patients using SABA alone who:
    - Are symptomatic >3x per week.
    - Wake 1x overnight per week.
    - Have suffered an exacerbation in the previous 2 years.
  - Side effects include oropharyngeal candidiasis and dysphonia.
  - In high-dose long-term use, may have impact on bone mineral density.
  - Potency of hydrofluoroalkane BDP is dependent upon inhaler brand and so must be prescribed by inhaler brand *not* generic name e.g. Clenil 400 mcg is equivalent to Qvar $200-300 mcg$.
- **Systemic Therapy:**
  - **Theophylline:**
    - Requires therapeutic drug monitoring.
    - Clearance is increased by smoking, alcohol and enzyme-inducing drugs and reduced by some antibiotics e.g. erythromycin.
    - Side effects include nausea, vomiting and abdominal discomfort, headache, malaise, tachycardia and fits.

- **Leukotriene-receptor antagonists (LTRA):** montelukast, zafirlukast.
  - Inhibit leukotriene receptors on smooth muscle preventing broncho-constriction, oedema and mucus production.
  - Used as an adjunct to inhaled therapy.
  - Can improve exercise induced bronchoconstriction.
  - May benefit those with NSAID/aspirin sensitivity.
- **Oral Steroids:**
  - Short courses (e.g. 40 mg prednisolone for 5 days) can be given during acute exacerbations.
  - Patients may occasionally require long-term steroid therapy.
  - Side effects include osteoporosis, immunosuppression, weight gain, hyperglycaemia and adrenal suppression.
  - Other immunosuppressants (cyclosporin, methotrexate) are rarely used now.
- **Anti IgE therapy (omalizumab)**
  - 2–4 weekly subcutaneous therapy in severe disease for patients with elevated total IgE to and sensitivity to a perennial aeroallergen.
  - Currently licensed by NICE for patients with 4 or more exacerbations per year requiring oral corticosteroid therapy or continuous corticosteroid use.
  - Non-compliance with existing treatments must be addressed prior to use.
  - Has a steroid sparing effect and can improve QoL and symptom score.
  - Side effects: Local skin irritation, anaphylaxis and serum sickness.
- **Anti-IL 5 therapy (mepolizumab, reslizumab, benralizumab)**
  - Either subcutaneous or intravenous monoclonal antibody therapy to target IL-5 – a cytokine involved in eosinophil migration and activation.
  - Criteria for use varies for each individual drug but in general licensed for patients with elevated blood eosinophil count who have a high exacerbation frequency and/or maintenance steroid use (dependent upon drug being used).

Stepwise management of asthma:

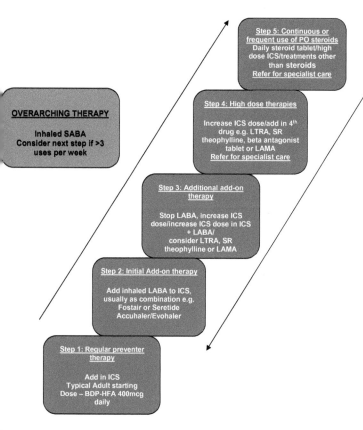

Figure 3.2 The stepwise control of asthma, adapted from BTS guidelines (see micro-ference). Move up and down the steps according to response to achieve optimum ntrol. SABA – short acting beta antagonist; ICS – inhaled corticosteroid; LABA – ng acting beta antagonist; LTRA – leukotriene receptor antagonist; SR theophylline – stained release theophylline.

Asthma action plans
- These form part of the self-management of asthma and should be given to all patients.
- They include clear written instructions on avoiding triggers, explaining medications, recognising worsening asthma symptoms and what action to take in this case.
- Advice should be clear, simple and tailored to the individual.
- Can reduce hospital admission frequency.

- **Difficult asthma**
  - Defined as persistent symptoms and/or frequent exacerbations despite treatment at step 4/5 of the stepwise approach (above).
  - Patients should be systematically evaluated for:
    - Confirmation of the asthma diagnosis.
    - Identification of the mechanism of the exacerbations/persisting symptoms.
    - Assessment of adherence to therapy.
    - Associated co-morbidities.
  - **Contributing factors:**
    - Poor adherence
    - Psychosocial factors
    - Smoking.
  - Management should facilitated by a multidisciplinary difficult asthma service.
  - Systemic monoclonal antibody therapy may be appropriate for patients with high corticosteroid use such as:
    - Anti-IgE treatment for atopic patients with perennial allergen exposure.
    - Anti-interleukin-5 treatment for eosinophilic disease.
  - Possible role for bronchial thermoplasty (thermoelectric current altering smooth muscle within endobronchial tree).

9. PROGNOSIS

- Persistent airway inflammation and remodelling can result in:
  - Fixed airway obstruction (becoming more like COPD).
  - Worsening lung function.
  - An acceleration in lung function decline occurs with frequent and severe exacerbations.
- Life expectancy is similar to the general population:
  - Approximately 1,300 people died from asthma in the UK in 2005.
  - Mortality is often associated with failure of the patient or staff to recognise the severity of the attack.
  - Asthma deaths are associated with 90% of preventable contributing factors e.g. non-adherence, poor inhaler technique and smoking.

3.1 ACUTE EXACERBATIONS OF ASTHMA

RECOGNITION OF ACUTE ASTHMA

- Severity of an acute exacerbation of asthma should be assessed using the criteria set out in Table 3.3.

Table 3.3 **Recognition of moderate severe and life-threatening asthma.**

	MODERATE EXACERBATION	ACUTE SEVERE ASTHMA	LIFE-THREATENING ASTHMA
PEFR	• 50–75% predicted/best	• 33–50% predicted/best	• <33% predicted/best
Clinical features	• Increasing symptoms • No features of acute severe asthma	• Resp. rate >25 • Heart rate >110 • SaO_2 ≥92% • Inability to complete sentence in one breath	• SaO_2 <92% • PaO_2 <8kPa • Normal or raised pCO_2 • Silent chest • Cyanosis • Poor respiratory effort • Bradycardia/ arrhythmia/ hypotension • Exhaustion • Confusion • Coma

MANAGEMENT OF ACUTE ASTHMA EXACERBATIONS

Initial management is carried out according to Figure 3.3:
Monitoring of the following should be carried out throughout:
- Peak expiratory flow rate:
  - Repeat $15 - 30$ minutes after starting treatment.
- Pulse oximetry
- Arterial blood gases:
  - If $SpO2 < 92\%$ initially.
  - Within 1 hour of starting treatment if initial $PaO_2 < 8kPa$, $PaCO_2$ normal/raised or patient deteriorates.

Respiratory Medicine

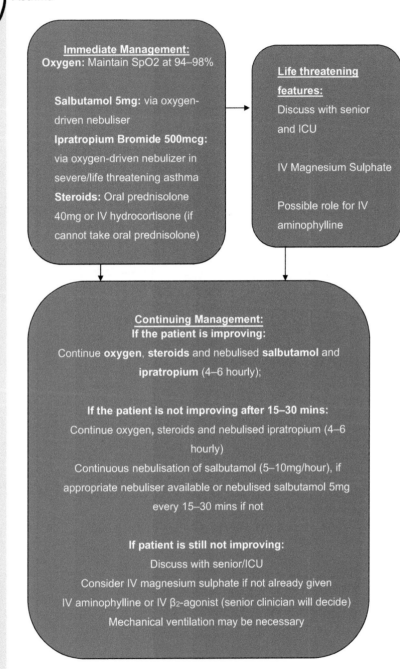

Figure 3.3 Management of an acute asthma exacerbation.

- **At discharge:**
  - Patients should have been on discharge medication for 12–24 hours.
  - Should be off nebulised therapy for minimum 24 hours.
  - Inhaler technique should have been checked.
  - PEFR > 75% in most cases with diurnal variation < 25%.
  - Issue with oral/inhaled steroids.
  - Provide written asthma action plan.
  - Address concomitant smoking.
  - Arrange follow-up:
    - With GP within 2 days.
    - At respiratory clinic within 4 weeks.

MICRO-case

You are an SHO working nights in A&E when a 20-year-old male student is brought in acutely short of breath. Initial examination and investigations reveal a respiratory rate of 33 with a heart rate of 117; however, SaO_2 is maintained at 94%. He tells you that he suffers with asthma and you begin management with oxygen, nebulised salbutamol, ipratropium, and oral prednisolone. His condition improves with this treatment and he is admitted to the ward where nebulised medication is administered every 4–6 hours until he is stabilised. After a further 24 hours without nebulised medication, he is stable on discharge medication and ready to go home. His inhaler technique is checked and found to be perfect, but further history taking reveals a worsening of his asthma over the last year or so: he is frequently woken by his symptoms and has struggled when playing football for the university team. A review of his prescription reveals that he is prescribed inhaled corticosteroids, LABA and SABA. He confesses that since starting university, he often forgets to take his medication, especially after a heavy night on the town. In addition, he is yet to register with the university GP so has missed several asthma review appointments.

Key Points

Severe asthma is suggested by:

- PEFR of 33–50% of predicted/best, inability to complete sentences, respiratory rate >25, heart rate > 110 but maintenance of O_2 saturation at > 92%.
- Life-threatening asthma is associated with:
  - Signs of exhaustion, such as a decreased respiratory effort, bradycardia, silent chest and decrease in O_2 saturations.

When managing difficult asthma, it is important to consider psychosocial factors and adherence to medication. Inhaler technique should be checked and an asthma action plan provided upon discharge from hospital.

Respiratory Medicine

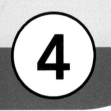

4 Chronic Obstructive Pulmonary Disease

1. DEFINITION

- Chronic obstructive pulmonary disease (COPD) is defined by non-reversible airflow limitation with variable combination of airway inflammation and parenchymal lung destruction.

2. EPIDEMIOLOGY

- It's estimated that there are ~1 million patients in England and Wales with diagnosed COPD.
- COPD is the fifth commonest cause of death in the UK.
- Diagnosis is usually in the seventh decade of life, and prevalence increases with age.

3. AETIOLOGY AND RISK FACTORS

- Cigarette smoking.
    - Most important risk factor.
- α1-Antitrypsin deficiency (see MICRO-Print).
- Air pollution.
- Occupational exposures:
    - Coal mining, concrete manufacturing, construction, foundry work, manufacturing, farming, transportation.
- Neonatal chronic lung disease (due to preterm birth) can result in emphysema.
- Repeated lower respiratory tract infections.
- History of pulmonary TB.

MICRO-print
α_1-Antitrypsin Deficiency
Autosomal recessive gene mutation in SERPINA gene on chromosome 14. Deficiency in α_1 antitrypsin leads to unopposed protease activity, especially neutrophil-derived elastases.

continued...

DOI: 10.1201/9781315113937-5

continued...

Diagnosed through a blood test – the lab will measure the absolute level of α1-antitrypsin, but will also assess the phenotype/genotype by isoelectric focussing where the protein migrates in a gel according to its isoelectric point or charge in a pH gradient. Normal A1AT is termed M, as it migrates toward the centre of the gel. Other variants are less functional and are termed A–L and N–Z, dependent on whether they run proximal or distal to the M band. Individuals inherit 2 copies of the gene and so the most common genotypes are:

- PiMM: 100% (normal).
- PiMS: 80% of normal serum level of A1AT.
- PiSS: 60% of normal serum level of A1AT.
- PiMZ: 60% of normal serum level of A1AT.
- PiSZ: 40% of normal serum level of A1AT.
- PiZZ: 10 − 15% (severe alpha-1 antitrypsin deficiency).

Individuals with one normal gene (M) are not at increased risk of disease but might need counselling on transmission to children. Those with two abnormal genes are at increased risk of:

- **Lung disease:** COPD.
- **Liver disease:** neonatal jaundice, hepatitis, cirrhosis, liver failure.

An IV replacement therapy has been developed but is not licensed in the UK.

4. PATHOPHYSIOLOGY

- Prolonged repeated exposure to noxious chemicals leads to increase in oxidative stress and results in adaptive changes within the lung.
- An exaggerated response to noxious substances may result in pathological changes, described below.
- Inflammation in COPD is mediated by neutrophils, macrophages, T-lymphocytes (particularly CD8 cells) and dendritic cells.
- Imbalance present between the action of proteases and anti-proteases (such as α1-antitrypsin).
    - Oxidative stress causes release of proteases from inflammatory cells promoting inactivation of antiproteases.
- Oxidative stress is pro-inflammatory and promotes mucus secretion.
- Chronic inflammation of the small airways, resulting in:
    - Fibrosis and remodelling.
    - Mucous cell hypertrophy.
    - Ciliary dysfunction and squamous metaplasia.
        - Difficulty expectorating inhaled pathogens, due to failure of the mucociliary escalator.

Respiratory Medicine

- Long-term airflow limitation:
  - In part due to the chronic inflammatory process in the conducting airways.
- Loss of elastic recoil in the airways results in airway collapse on expiration:
  - Results in air trapping and hyperinflation of the lungs.
  - Hyperinflation reduces the inspiratory capacity and functional residual capacity.
  - This causes shortness of breath on exertion.
- Ventilation-perfusion mismatch:
  - Causes hypoxaemia with or without hypercapnia.

5. CLINICAL FEATURES

- **Symptoms**
  - Productive cough.
  - Wheeze.
  - Breathlessness, particularly on exertion (see MICRO-Facts mMRC dyspnoea score).
  - Frequent exacerbations, often caused by respiratory infection.
- **Signs**
  - **Mild disease:**
    - May be none.
    - Wheeze.
  - **In severe disease:**
    - Tachypnoea.
    - Prolonged expiratory phase.
    - Use of accessory muscles of respiration.
    - Pursing of lips.
    - Intercostal indrawing.
    - Hyperinflated chest and decreased chest expansion.
    - Signs of cor pulmonale in late disease.
    - Low BMI.

MICRO-facts

The mMRC (Modified Medical Research Council) Dyspnoea Scale is used to assess the degree of baseline functional disability due to dyspnoea.

Respiratory Medicine

SCORE	SYMPTOMS
0	Breathless only with strenuous exercise.
1	Short of breath when hurrying or walking up a hill.
2	Slower than most people of same age on level because of breathlessness, or have to stop for breath when walking at own pace on the level.
3	Stop for breath after walking ~100 m or after a few minutes at own pace on the level.
4	Too breathless to leave house/breathless when dressing.

MICRO-references
British Thoracic Society (BTS) NICE guideline for COPD (updated 2019), available at:
www.nice.org.uk/guidance/ng115

6. INVESTIGATIONS

- **Spirometry:**
  - Spirometry should be performed for diagnosis in all patients with suspected COPD.
  - A diagnosis of airflow obstruction can be made if the FEV_1/FVC ratio is less than 0.7 (70%). See Chapter 1: Clinical assessment.
  - If $FEV_1 > 80\%$, appropriate symptoms are required to confirm the diagnosis.
  - Severity of airflow obstruction is classified as in Table 4.1.

Table 4.1 **Severity of COPD.**

STAGE	SEVERITY	POST BRONCHODILATOR FEV_1/FVC	POST BRONCHODILATOR FEV_1 (% OF PREDICTED)
1	Mild	<0.7	≥80
2	Moderate	<0.7	50–79
3	Severe	<0.7	30–49
4	Very Severe	<0.7	<30 or <50 with respiratory failure

Respiratory Medicine

- Unlike asthma, COPD does not usually demonstrate much reversibility.
  - A diagnosis of COPD should be reconsidered if there is a large (>400 mL) response to inhaled therapy and/or oral prednisolone (See Table 4.2).
- **Imaging:**
  - **Chest X-ray**
    - To exclude other lung diseases.
    - Often normal in early stages of the disease.
    - Advanced COPD may have the following features on chest X-ray (see Figure 4.1):
      - Hyperinflated lungs
      - Flattened diaphragm
      - Hyperlucent lungs
      - Central pulmonary artery dilatation
      - Bullae.

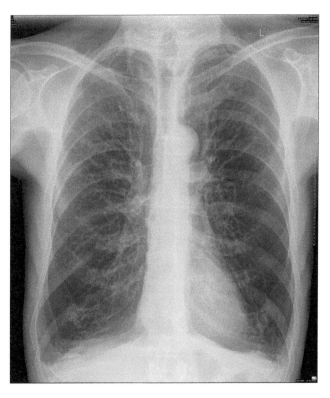

Figure 4.1 Chest X-ray of a patient with COPD. The X-ray shows that the lungs are hyperinflated and the diaphragms are flattened.

- **CT scan:**
  - This is more effective for detecting pathological changes such as emphysema but is not routinely performed (See Figure 4.2).

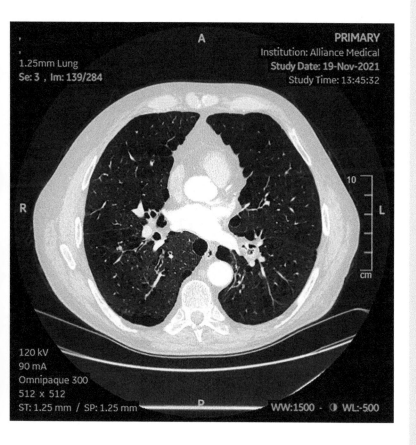

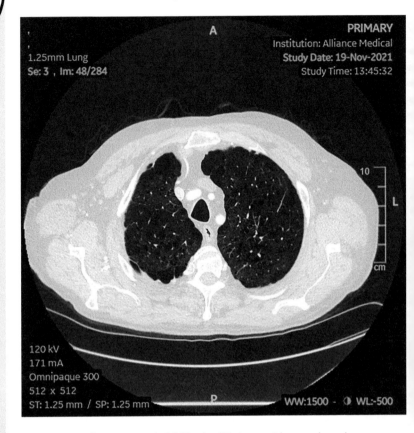

Figure 4.2 CT of a patient with COPD; the CT shows widespread emphysema.

- **Blood tests:**
  - **FBC:** May show polycythaemia secondary to persistent hypoxaemia in severe disease.
- **ECG and echocardiogram:**
  - Used to determine presence of cor pulmonale.
- **Carbon monoxide transfer factor (T_{Lco}):**
  - This measures the diffusion capacity of gases from the alveoli to the capillaries.
  - A reduced diffusion capacity is a feature of emphysema but can be seen in other conditions.
- **Sputum culture:**
  - This can be considered if the patient presents with an infective episode.
- **Pulse oximetry:**
  - Pulse oximetry can be performed to screen patients for oxygen therapy (see below).

7. DIFFERENTIAL DIAGNOSIS

- Asthma (see Table 4.2)
- Bronchiectasis
- Lung cancer
- Congestive cardiac failure
- Tuberculosis
- Interstitial lung disease.

Table 4.2 **Differentiating between COPD and Asthma.**

	COPD	ASTHMA
Age	>35	Any age, often younger
Cough	Productive, persistent	Non-productive, variable
Smoking	Nearly always	Possible
Breathlessness	Progressive	Variable
Diurnal variability	Not usual	Worse at night/early in the morning
Reversibility	Not reversible with inhaled bronchodilators	Reversible with inhaled bronchodilators
Eczema/allergic rhinitis	Possible	Common
Family history	Not usual	Common, as is a family history of eczema/allergic rhinitis

8. MANAGEMENT

- **Smoking cessation:**
  - This is one of the most important components of COPD management and should be encouraged at every opportunity (see chapter on smoking and the lung).
- **Pharmacological management:**
  - **Inhaled therapy** (see Figure 4.1):
  - **Short-acting beta agonists:** e.g. salbutamol, terbutaline.
  - **Short-acting muscarinic antagonists:** e.g. ipratropium bromide (rarely used now as long-acting drugs more effective).
  - **Long-acting beta agonists:** e.g. salmeterol, formoterol.
  - **Long-acting muscarinic antagonists:** e.g. tiotropium, aclidinium.
  - **Combination long-acting beta agonist and long-acting muscarinic antagonists:** e.g. Spioloto (tiotropium and olodaterol), Duaklir (formoterol and aclidinium). Can improve symptoms and reduce exacerbations. Currently in use but not within present NICE algorithm.

Respiratory Medicine

- **Combination long-acting beta agonist and corticosteroid inhalers:** e.g. Seretide (salmeterol and beclamethasone) and Symbicort (formoterol and budesonide), primarily reserved for patients with increased exacerbation frequency and reduced lung function.
- **Inhaled corticosteroids are not licensed in monotherapy:** use of corticosteroids are linked with increased risk of pneumonia, skin bruising, reduced bone mineral density, oral candidiasis.
- **Oral therapy:**
- **Theophylline:** a non-specific phosphodiesterase inhibitor which acts as a bronchodilator.
  - It also has an anti-inflammatory effect and increases mucociliary clearance.
  - A narrow therapeutic index, drug interactions and adverse effects limit its use, e.g. nausea, palpitations, arrhythmias.
- **Oral corticosteroids:** Used for their anti-inflammatory effects.
  - Little evidence to support their role in long-term use.
  - Long-term steroid therapy is associated with systemic adverse effects.
- **Mucolytics:** Reduce the viscosity of secretions and facilitate expectoration.
  - Carbocysteine and mecysteine hydrochloride are licensed for this use.
  - For use if patients find symptomatic benefit after fixed period trial.
- **Pulmonary rehabilitation:**
  - Includes physical training, disease education, nutritional, psychological and behavioural interventions.
  - It should be offered to all appropriate patients.
  - Not suitable for patients with recent myocardial infarction or unstable angina, or who have locomotor difficulties that preclude exercise.
- **Nutrition:**
  - Patients with abnormal BMIs should be referred for dietetic advice.
  - Nutritional supplementation may be required.
- **Long-term oxygen therapy (LTOT):**
  - Offered to patients with respiratory failure. In general decisions about LTOT should not be made in a stable state and not immediately after an exacerbation).
    - $P_aO_2 < 7.3 \ kPa$
    - $P_aO_2 < 8 \ kPa$ and one of the following features:
      - Secondary polycythaemia
      - Peripheral oedema
      - Nocturnal hypoxaemia
      - Pulmonary hypertension.

- **Ambulatory oxygen:**
  - Offered to patients who desaturate on exertion if they are slow to recover to baseline and if it can be shown to improve their exercise tolerance.
- **Lung volume reduction (LVR):**
  - Patients with significant emphysema and hyperinflation on lung function testing may gain improvement in breathlessness and exercise tolerance from reducing the volume of lung tissue by "removing" the most diseased areas of the lung. LVR can be done by surgical resection, or by collapsing segments/lobes by occluding airways through insertion of one way valves. Patients must have stopped smoking and completed pulmonary rehabilitation. Specialist assessment by an LVR MDT is required.
- **Non-invasive ventilation (NIV):**
  - Some patients with persistent stable hypercapnic (type 2) respiratory failure may benefit from domiciliary NIV, which has not been shown to reduce mortality but does appear to reduce frequency of hospital admission. It can also be used to support delivery of LTOT in such patients.
- **Lung transplantation:**
  - An option for younger patients who have no other major co-morbidities.

9. COMPLICATIONS

- Pulmonary hypertension with signs of cor pulmonale.
- Respiratory failure.

10. PROGNOSIS

- COPD has a variable prognosis.
- Over time, dyspnoea and frequency of infective exacerbations increase.
- Patients may become oxygen dependant.
- The **BODE Index** (see MICRO-Facts box) is used as a measure of disease severity and therefore prognosis.

MICRO-facts

The BODE Index Is a Prognostic Indicator

- **B**MI
- (Airflow) **O**bstruction
- **D**yspnoea (see Table 4.2)
- **E**xercise capacity

continued...

Respiratory Medicine

continued...

VARIABLE	POINTS			
	0	**1**	**2**	**3**
Body Mass Index	>21	≤21		
Obstruction: FEV$_1$ (% Predicted)	≥65	50–64	36–49	≤35
Dyspnoea: mMRC Dyspnoea Scale (see below)	0–1	2	3	4
Exercise Tolerance: 6-minute walk test in metres	≥350	250–349	150–249	≤149

- **Negative prognostic factors:**
  - Very low weight.
  - Low exercise tolerance.
  - Increased breathlessness with activity.
  - Frequent exacerbations.
  - Requiring multiple episodes of intubation and mechanical ventilation.
- **Factors that improve survival:**
  - Smoking cessation.
  - Oxygen supplementation.

4.1 ACUTE EXACERBATIONS OF COPD

1. RECOGNITION

- Worsening dyspnoea.
- Increased cough.
- Increased sputum volume.
- Change in sputum colour.
- Increased wheeze or chest tightness.
- Reduced exercise tolerance.
- Increased fatigue.
- Marked respiratory distress: tachypnoea, cyanosis, confusion, peripheral oedema.

2. PATHOPHYSIOLOGY

- Most often caused by acute respiratory viral/bacterial infection.
- Similar presentation can be seen with pulmonary embolism, heart failure or lung cancer.

3. INVESTIGATIONS

- FBC, U&E.
- Pulse oximetry, and consider ABG if hypoxic.
- Blood cultures if pyrexial.
- CXR.
- ECG.

MICRO-case

You are working in a respiratory outpatient clinic when a 64-year-old ex-miner comes to see you after a GP referral. As he walks into the consultation room, you notice that he's markedly out of breath. He tells you that for the last few years he's been becoming gradually more out of breath and now struggles to do his own cleaning and shopping. He cannot keep up with friends of the same age and often stops to catch his breath when walking alone. In addition, he has a persistent cough which brings up yellowy phlegm. In the last few years he's had a number of chest infections which he's struggled to shake off. He has smoked since he was 14, which you calculate as 50 pack-years. Spirometry reveals an FEV_1/FVC ratio of 0.65 and an FEV_1 which is 50% of predicted. You weigh and measure him and determine that his BMI is 19.5. You emphasise the importance of giving up smoking and commence him on inhaled therapy and recommend that he book a GP appointment for his annual influenza vaccination. You refer him for pulmonary rehabilitation, where he is found to be able to walk 200 m in 6 minutes. From the information you have obtained, you calculate that his BODE index is 5.

Key Points

- The BODE index is an important prognostic indicator.
- It is scored out of 10, with a higher score associated with increased mortality.
- The four components are BMI, (Airflow) Obstruction, Dyspnoea and Exercise capacity.
- A history of smoking is the most important risk factor and one of the first elements which should be addressed in managing the condition.
- Influenza vaccine should be offered to those with COPD (see also Chapter 2: Respiratory Infections).

---

4. MANAGEMENT

- **Assess whether admission to hospital is necessary:**
  - Severe respiratory distress or poor condition.
  - Unable to cope at home.
  - Already on LTOT.

  - Changes on CXR.
  - Impaired consciousness/confusion.
  - Associated co-morbidity.
  - $SaO_2 < 90\%$, $P_aO_2 < 7kPa$, $pH < 7.35$.
- **High-dose short-acting bronchodilators:** salbutamol or ipratropium bromide.
- **Oral steroids:** prednisolone for 5–7 days.
- **Antibiotic therapy:** with sputum colour change and increase in volume, or signs of consolidation.
- **Nicotine replacement therapy:** if an active smoker.
- **Oxygen therapy:** in the absence of ABG results, titrate SpO2 to $88 - 92\%$ initially.
- **Physiotherapy:** helpful in some cases to aid sputum clearance; used in conjunction with mucolytics such as carbocisteine or nebulised saline.
- **Non-invasive ventilation (NIV):** if persistent hypercapnic respiratory failure with acidosis.
- **Pulmonary rehabilitation:** following recovery from the acute episode.

Lung Malignancy

5.1 PRIMARY LUNG MALIGNANCY

1. EPIDEMIOLOGY

- The rate of lung cancer in men and women is 87 and 67, respectively, per 100,000 per year.
- It is the commonest cause of cancer related death in both men and women worldwide.
    - Third commonest cause of death in the UK.
    - Five-year survival rate is dependent upon histology and stage of disease but is generally poor.
- The incidence of lung cancer in the UK has been declining in both men and women and has been attributed to decreased rates of smoking.
- Further epidemiological statistics are available at the Cancer Research UK website: www.cancerresearchuk.org/health-professional/cancer-statistics/statistics-by-cancer-type/lung-cancer

2. AETIOLOGY AND RISK FACTORS

- Cigarette smoking (including passive smoking) accounts for around 70% of lung cancers.
- Risk factors:
    - Tobacco smoking.
    - Environmental tobacco exposure.
    - Air pollution.
    - Radon exposure and other forms of ionising radiation.
    - Asbestos exposure.
    - Occupational exposure: arsenic, nickel, chromium or petroleum products.
    - Pulmonary fibrosis.
    - Chronic obstructive pulmonary disease (COPD).
    - Human immunodeficiency virus (HIV)/acquired immunodeficiency syndrome (AIDS).

DOI: 10.1201/9781315113937-6

> **MICRO-print**
> Most tumours arise from the bronchi close to the hilum. As a result, most malignancies of the lung will involve the upper lobe or main bronchus.

3. PATHOPHYSIOLOGY

- Lung cancers are usually divided histologically, into small cell lung cancer (SCLC) and non-small cell lung cancer (NSCLC), and the latter can be further subdivided. A precise histopathological diagnosis is important due to general differences in principles of management and prognosis.
- **NSCLC:**
  - NSCLC accounts for 85% of primary lung malignancy and is further divided into a number of subtypes, dependent on histological appearance and the cells of origin (Table 5.1).
  - Sometimes the NSCLC subtype is well differentiated, and it is easy for the pathologist to recognise, but often an immunohistochemical panel will be needed to classify.

Table 5.1 **Subtypes of NSCLC.**

TYPES	% NSCLC	PATHOLOGY	CLINICAL FEATURES
Adenocarcinoma	38	Originates from mucous cells in bronchial epithelium. Associated with asbestos exposure and more common in non-smokers.	Arises peripherally. Early metastatic spread to bone and brain.
Squamous cell carcinoma (large cell neuroendocrine carcinoma)	20	Originates from squamous epithelial lining of the bronchi. Subset of neuroendocrine lung tumours. Lesions are cavitating.	Lesions involve the central airways. They tend to grow quickly and are locally invasive but metastasise late in the disease course.

(Continued)

Table 5.1 (*continued*) Subtypes of NSCLC.

TYPES	% NSCLC	PATHOLOGY	CLINICAL FEATURES
Carcinoid tumours	7	Originating from neuroendocrine tissue. Often includes Kulchitsky cells.	Can cause carcinoid syndrome. The tumour is usually extremely vascular and prone to bleeding.
Large cell	5	Poorly differentiated cell, of uncertain histological origin, named for their excess cytoplasm and large nuclei. Almost a diagnosis of exclusion as no features of other types of NSCLC.	Often presents as a large peripheral mass. High risk for early metastatic spread.
Minimally invasive adenocarcinoma	<4	Can be considered adenocarcinoma-in-situ, re-classified in 2011: • Pre-invasive atypical adenomatous hyperplasia (pre-malignant). • Adenocarcinoma in situ (AIS) <3 cm, lacks invasion and distribution is restricted to alveolar structures (so-called lepidic growth pattern). • Minimally invasive AIS, displays invasion ≤5 mm.	Non-invasive lesion, completely curable by adequate surgical resection. Lesion can progress to a sub-type of adenocarcinoma if left untreated.

- There are a small proportion of NSCLC that are unable to be identified and classified into these main subtypes.
- Immunohistochemistry can also be used to determine if an adenocarcinoma has originated in the lung or metastasised from elsewhere

Respiratory Medicine

(e.g. TTF-1 positivity is strongly suggestive of primary lung adenocarcinoma).

- Since the introduction of immunotherapy treatment (see below), an immunohistochemical analysis for PDL-1 expression will usually be undertaken.
- Many adenocarcinomas and some other tumours will have "driver mutations" that can be targeted by specific small molecule drugs (e.g. epidermal growth factor receptor (EGFR), anaplastic lymphoma kinase (ALK) and ROS proto-oncogene 1 (ROS-1). IT is now increasingly common for the whole tumour genome and RNA expression to be analysed through next-generation sequencing (NGS) to detect all potential driver mutations.

- **SCLC:**
  - SCLC (also called oat cell carcinoma) accounts for approximately 15% of all lung cancers and is more closely related to smoking than other lung cancers.
    - Originates from Kulchitsky cells, part of the amine precursor uptake and decarboxylation (APUD) endocrine system.
    - It is sometimes called oat cell carcinoma because of its histological appearance.
    - These tumours usually arise centrally with mediastinal involvement.
    - They are highly aggressive, with two-thirds of patients having distant metastases at presentation.

- **Metastases:**
  - The primary lung cancers can spread to distant sites, most commonly:
    - Brain
    - Bone
    - Liver
    - Adrenal glands.

4. CLINICAL FEATURES

- Risk factors in the history for lung malignancy:
  - Male sex.
  - Age >50 yrs.
  - History of smoking (first- or second-hand exposure).
  - Asbestos exposure.
  - Previous cancer (either locally or elsewhere).
  - Dyspnoea.
- Symptoms and signs are shown in Figure 5.1. These may be non-specific, related to the primary tumour itself, due to metastatic spread (commonest sites brain, bone, liver adrenals) or sometimes caused by a paraneoplastic syndrome.

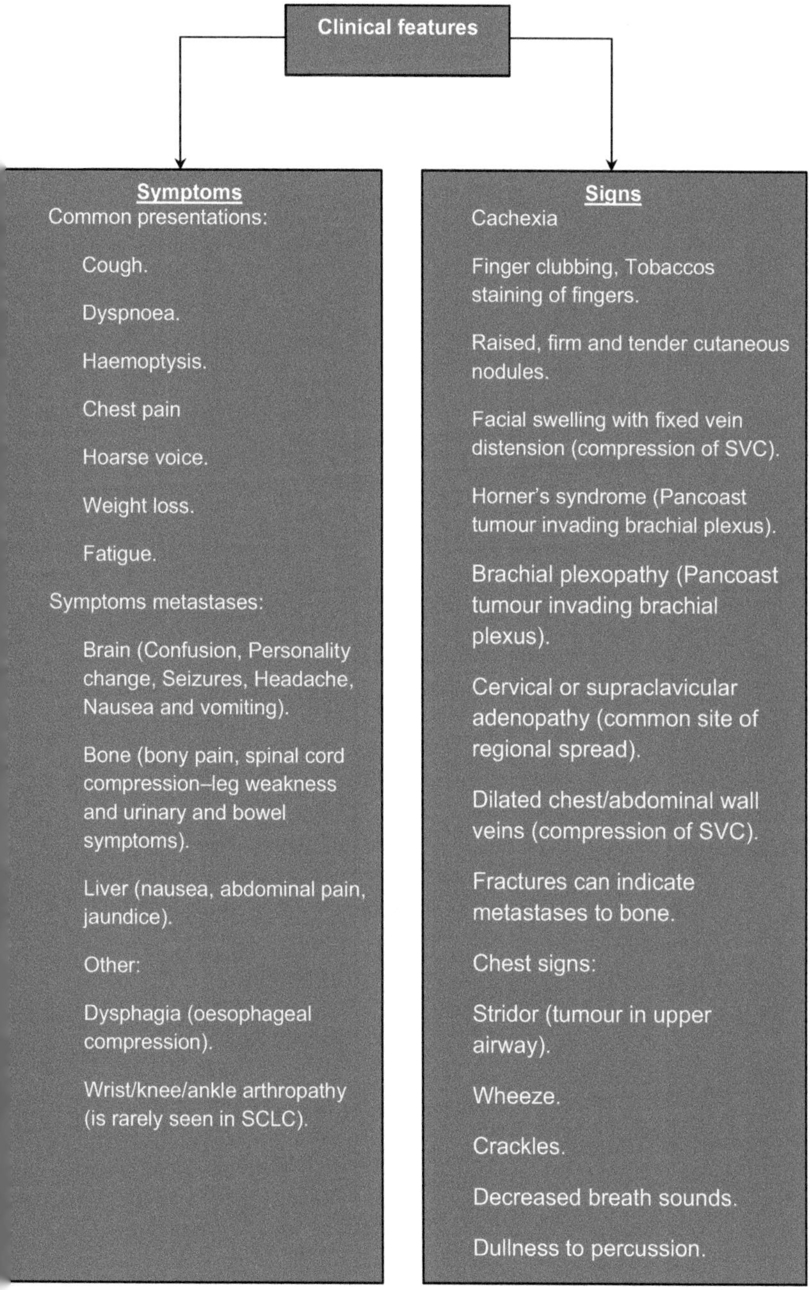

igure 5.1 Clinical features of lung malignancy.

MICRO-facts

Horner's syndrome is a rare condition. It is a triad of physical signs which are the manifestation of the disruption of the sympathetic innervation of the eye. It can be caused by a wide variety of disease processes. The triad of signs are:

Ipsilateral partial ptosis
Ipsilateral miosis
Hemifacial ipsilateral anhidrosis.

Horner's syndrome can be caused by Pancoast's tumour of lung and can form part of a constellation of symptoms and signs known as **Pancoast's syndrome.** In addition to Horner's syndrome, these include:

Shoulder and arm pain.
Wasting of the intrinsic muscles of the hand.
Paraesthesia in medial side of the arm.
Hoarse voice (due to unilateral recurrent laryngeal nerve palsy).
Oedema of the arm.

5. PARANEOPLASTIC SYNDROMES

- Paraneoplastic syndromes result from either local secretion of hormone/cytokines from the tumour itself or an immune response directed against the tumour.
- They may be reversible with adequate treatment of the cancer.
- There are a number of paraneoplastic effects that are of importance in lung cancer:
- **Syndrome of inappropriate antidiuretic hormone (SIADH):**
  - Excess antidiuretic hormone (ADH) secretion, leading to impaired water excretion and a subsequent state of euvolaemic hypotonic hyponatraemia.
    - Consequently, severe neurological symptoms can ensue:
      - Altered mental state
      - Nausea and vomiting
      - Seizures
      - Coma.
    - Treatment of SIADH due to paraneoplastic syndrome includes:
      - Fluid restriction.
      - Democycline.
      - Vasopressin receptor antagonist e.g. desmopressin.
      - Treatment of underlying cancer.
      - In cases of unwell patients with very low serum sodium levels, intravenous hypertonic saline can be administered carefully.

- ○ Note: Rapid correction of serum sodium can result in central pontine myelinolysis (CPM).
- ○ To prevent CPM hyponatraemia should not be corrected at a rate greater than 10 mmol/L/24hr.

Hypercalcaemia:

- Can be due to ectopic secretion of parathyroid hormone release or osteolytic bone disease (bony metastases).
  - – Patients with hypercalcaemia due to malignancy have a poorer prognosis.
  - – Clinical features:
    - ○ Muscle weakness.
    - ○ Constipation and abdominal pain.
    - ○ Anorexia, nausea and vomiting.
    - ○ Stone formation e.g. nephrocalcinosis.
    - ○ Bone pain.
    - ○ Pancreatitis.
    - ○ Cardiac arrhythmias (shortened QT interval).
    - ○ Coma.
  - – Treatment should be initiated by a specialist and may include:
    - ○ Normal saline infusion (approximately 3L/24hr depending on cardiovascular status).
    - ○ Bisphosphonates e.g. zoledronic acid.
    - ○ Addition of loop diuretic in resistant cases.
    - ○ Gallium nitrate.
    - ○ Plicamycin: occasionally used.

Hypertrophic pulmonary osteoarthropathy (Bamberger-Marie syndrome):

- Combination of clubbing and periostitis.
  - – It is more closely associated with adenocarcinoma than other lung malignancies.
  - – More common in NSCLC than SCLC.
  - – Defined by osseus proliferation resulting in expansion of the long bones of upper and lower limbs.
    - ○ Bone pain can occur.
    - ○ Joints are often swollen and tender.
  - – The condition can be reversed if lung mass is removed or the vagus nerve is severed.

Lambert-Eaton syndrome:

- Rare autoimmune disorder of the neuromuscular junction: it is usually due to SCLC.
  - – Characterised by the presence of circulating auto-antibodies against voltage gated calcium channels.

- ○ Impairs neuromuscular transmission by inhibiting inward calcium current to the neuron.
- ○ Thus preventing release of acetylcholine into the synaptic cleft.
- – It causes a number of symptoms due to its effect at the neuromuscular junction:
  - ○ Weakness
  - ○ Dry mouth
  - ○ Ptosis
  - ○ Impotence
  - ○ Dysphagia
  - ○ Dysarthria
  - ○ Diplopia
  - ○ Orthostatic hypotension.
- – Most importantly, the underlying malignancy should be treated, but there are number of additional treatment options:
  - ○ Amifampridine +/- pyridostigmine.
  - ○ Immunomodulators e.g. prednisolone.
  - ○ Plasma exchange or intravenous immunoglobulins (IVIG).
- – Intubation and mechanical ventilation may be needed if there is severe respiratory or bulbar weakness.

6. DIFFERENTIAL DIAGNOSIS

- When a patient initially presents symptoms may be non-specific, and the differential diagnosis may include:
  - Pneumonia/lower respiratory tract infection (LRTI).
  - Metastatic tumour (non-thoracic primary).
  - TB or other infectious process.
  - Sarcoidosis.
  - Rheumatoid arthritis (rheumatoid nodules/Caplan's syndrome).
  - Wegener's granulomatosis.
  - Hamartoma.
  - Arteriovenous malformation.
  - Amyloidosis.
  - Cryptogenic organising pneumonia (COP).
  - Lymphoma.
  - Bronchogenic cyst.
- Note: If lung malignancy is suspected, it should be generally confirmed or excluded as a matter of urgency before other differentials are considered. However, in some cases radiological surveillance may be appropriate to avoid potentially unnecessary invasive investigation.

Respiratory Medicine

7. INVESTIGATIONS

- Initially investigations will almost always include:
  - Chest X-ray postero-anterior (PA) (see Figure 5.2):
    - May detect mass, pulmonary nodule, hilar and mediastinal lymph-adenopathy, pleural effusion or lung collapse. Lateral views are rarely used.

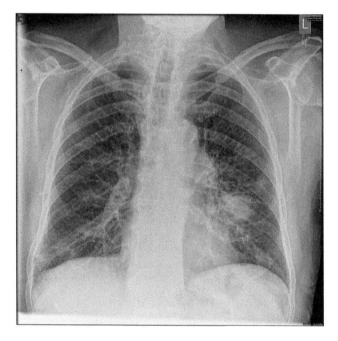

Figure 5.2 CXR of patient with lung cancer; there is a circular opacity in the perihilar region of the left lung that indicates a mass.

  - Contrast enhanced chest and abdominal computed tomography (CT):
    - Used to show size and location of primary tumour, as well as assessing for metastases thereby providing staging investigation (see Figure 5.3).
    - Sputum cytology:
    - Detects malignant cells in sputum but diagnostic yield is very poor and it is rarely used.

Respiratory Medicine

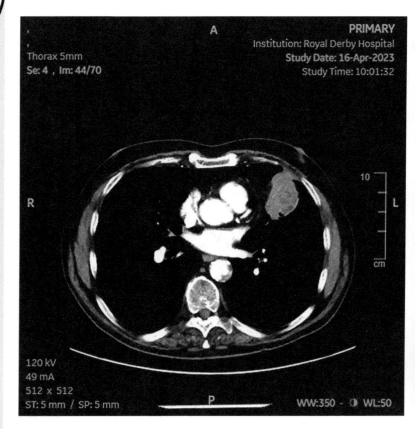

Figure 5.3 CT chest of a patient with lung cancer; a circular opacity is seen in the left lung.

MICRO-facts

- Generally investigations of suspected lung cancer are to answer the "3 Ws".
- Where is it? – the extent or stage of the cancer which will determine prognosis and treatment options
- What is it? – a biopsy needed to determine if this is lung cancer and what is the pathological subtype?
- What do we do about it? – the fitness of the patient in terms of co-morbidities, respiratory/cardiac function and performance status, which as well as the above will influence the treatment options.

Respiratory Medicine

- There are a number of further investigations that can be considered to aid diagnosis and staging. Tests which provide both (e.g. EBUS of mediastinal lymph nodes) in a single test are preferred (see Table 5.2).

Table 5.2 **Investigations in suspected lung malignancy.**

INVESTIGATIONS	
Bronchoscopy	Used to visualise and biopsy endobronchial lesions. Offer to those with central lesion if CT nodal staging does not influence treatment.
CT chest, abdomen, and pelvis	Provides staging information, especially if lung malignancy might be secondary.
Thoracic magnetic resonance imaging (MRI)	Should not be routinely performed. Can be considered to access extent of disease in patients with a superior sulcus tumour or if bone/adrenal metastases are suspected.
PET (positron emission tomography)-CT	Should be offered to every patient who is potential suitable for treatment with curative intent. Used to accurately assess the presence of local, regional and distant disease (See Figure 5.4).
Brain imaging	Indicated if symptoms suggest brain metastases, but also in asymptomatic stage II/III patients being considered for curative-intent treatment.
Ultrasound	May be used to assess chest wall invasion, to assess liver masses, or to assist in biopsy procedures (e.g. pleural fluid aspiration).
Thoracoscopy or VATS (video-assisted thorascopic surgery)	Allows direct visualisation of the pleura, useful in the assessment of potentially malignant pleural effusion. VATS can also be used to biopsy hilar lymph nodes.
EBUS-guided TBNA	Endobronchial ultrasound guided transbronchial needle biopsy (EBUS-guided TBNA) should be offered for paratracheal and peribronchial intra-parenchymal lesions, or if there is an intermediate or high probability of mediastinal malignancy. With central adenopathy > 2 cm, TBNA minus ultrasound guidance can be offered.
Physiological assessment	Cardiac echo and lung function testing are usually required in patients who are anticipated to undergo curative-intent treatment (especially if surgical).

Respiratory Medicine

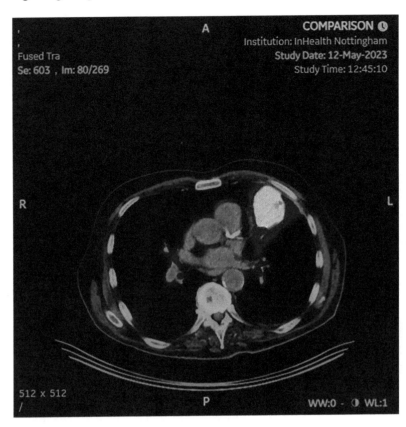

Figure 5.4 PET-CT chest; image is of the same patient as Figure 5.3 and shows an enhancing lesion where the cancer is in the left chest.

- Biopsy is considered the gold standard for diagnosis; pathological diagnosis of lung cancer is the only method widely accepted.

8. STAGING

- Primary lung malignancy (both NSCLC and SCLC) is staged using the TNM (tumour, node, metastases) system (see Figures 5.5, 5.6 and 5.7).
- The stagings are then grouped, these grouping are used to decide on intervention and estimate prognosis (See Table 5.3).

MICRO-facts

The WHO performance status (PS) classification is used to estimate the overall functional status of patients which in turn often guides treatment options. In general, patients with PS 3–4 will only be suitable for best supportive (palliative care).

- 0: able to carry out all normal activity without restriction.
- 1: restricted in strenuous activity but ambulatory and able to carry out light work.
- 2: ambulatory and capable of all self-care but unable to carry out any work activities; up and about more than 50% of waking hours.
- 3: symptomatic and in a chair or in bed for greater than 50% of the day but not bedridden.
- 4: completely disabled; cannot carry out any self-care; totally confined to bed or chair.

- **Tumour:**

T0: No evidence of primary tumour
Tis: Carcinoma in situ

T1:
Diameter ≤ 3cm.
T1a(mi) Minimally Invasive Adenocarcinoma
T1a1cm
T1b>1cm2cm
T1c>2cm3cm

T2:
Diameter ≥3cm but <5cm
Any of the following features:

Involves the main bronchus with no carina involvement

Invasion of visceral pleura.

Obstructive pneumonitis or atelectasis extending to hilar region

T2a Tumour >3cm but ≤4cm
T2b Tumour >4cm but ≤5cm

T3:
Tumour >5cm and ≤7cm
Additional satellite nodules within same lobe
Directly invasion of:-

Chest wall.

Phrenic nerve.

Parietal percardium.

T4:
Satellite lesions within ipsilateral lung outside on original lobe.
Invasion of mediastinal organs:

Oesophagus.

Trachea.

Great vessels.

Heart.

Mediastinum

Vertebral body

Figure 5.5 Staging of lung tumour: TNM system.

Respiratory Medicine

- **Node involvement:**

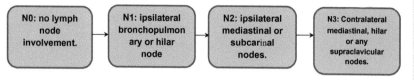

Figure 5.6 Staging of nodal involvement: TNM system.

- **Metastatic involvement:**

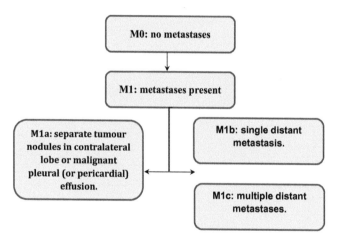

Figure 5.7 Staging of metastases: TNM system.

Respiratory Medicine

Table 5.3 **Staging of NSCLC to determine prognosis and treatment.**

STAGE GROUPINGS OF NSCLC	TNM STAGES
Occult carcinoma	Tx N0 M0
Stage 0	Tis N0 M0
Stage IA1	T1a N0 M0
	T1a (mis) N0 M0
Stage IA2	T1b N0 M0
Stage IA3	T1c N0 M0
Stage IB	T2a N0 M0
Stage IIA	T2b N0 M0
Stage IIB	T1a-c N1 M0 T2a-b N1 M0 T3 N0 M0
Stage IIIA	T1–3 N2 M0 T3 N1 M0 T4 N0–1 M0
Stage IIIB	T1–2 N3 M0 T-3 N2 M0
Stage IIIC	T3–4 N3 M0
Stage IVA	ANY M1a or M1b
Stage IVB	Any M1c

- The TNM stagings are then grouped, for intervention and prognosis.

9. MANAGEMENT

- The range of treatment options for lung cancer have dramatically expanded over the past decade and depend greatly on disease stage, tumour subtype and patient fitness.
- All new diagnoses of lung cancer should be discussed at a multi-disciplinary meeting so that the most appropriate options can be recommended.
- **General principles:**
  - **Breaking bad news should ideally be done in the presence of a specialist nurse.**
  - Advise patients that they should stop smoking and offer referral to smoking cessation services.

- Refer early to dietetics if there is weight loss, to rehab services if functionally impaired and to palliative care if advanced disease with symptoms.
- Patients will enter a surveillance programme after competing primary treatment to monitor for complications, and to detect new or recurrent cancer as early as possible.
- The main treatment modalities are surgery, systemic anti-cancer therapy (SACT) and radiotherapy.
- Surgery rarely used in SCLC – usually involves chemotherapy (and radiotherapy if curative-intent).
- SACT includes traditional cytotoxic chemotherapy (such as cisplatin and pemetrexed), immunotherapy (such as pembrolizumab) and targeted therapies such as tyrosine kinase inhibitors (e.g. Osimertinib).
- Radiotherapy regimens include stereotactic ablative body radiotherapy (SABR) which can accurately deliver high doses to a tumour and minimise toxicity providing an alternative to surgery, especially in older and less fit patients with small tumours.

Curative-intent treatment:

- Stage IIIA and below may be curable with single modality (surgery, radiotherapy), or multi-modality (chemo-radiotherapy) treatments.
- SACT may be given before (neo-adjuvant) or after (adjuvant) surgery to reduce risk of relapse.

Palliative-intent treatment:

- Aim is to prolong life and palliate symptoms. Important that side effects of treatment should overall reduce and not add to the burden of symptoms.
- Choice of first-line SACT depends on whether there is a driver mutation (offer targeted therapy), whether there is high PL-1 expression (offer immunotherapy), or neither (offer chemotherapy).
- Some treatments (e.g. targeted therapy) continue until relapse; others are given as a course and then patients monitored. Patients will often undergo multiple lines of treatment if their PS allows.
- Palliative radiotherapy can be useful for local symptoms such as bone pain or haemoptysis.
- Treatment of SCLC is not as successful as that for NSCLC: relapse is more common, however, it is usually very chemotherapy responsive.

0. COMPLICATIONS

SVCO (Superior vena cava obstruction):

- Lung cancer is the most common cause of superior vena cava obstruction.
  - It is usually due to mediastinal adenopathy or medial extension of a right upper lobe tumour.

Respiratory Medicine

- Blood flow from the face and arms is prevented from returning to the heart, resulting in the following presentation:
  - Facial and upper extremity oedema.
  - Dyspnoea.
  - Orthopnoea.
  - Cough.
  - Facial plethora upon raising arms above the head (Pemberton's sign)
  - Distension of superficial neck, chest wall and upper abdominal veins.
  - Headache.
  - Syncope.
- Treatment is directed primarily at the underlying pathology.
  - High-dose steroids are often given as a temporary measure but have limited impact.
  - SVC stent insertion can provide rapid relief of symptoms but risks complications such as stent thrombosis.
  - For patients with NSCLC radiotherapy can be considered.
  - For SCLC, primary chemotherapy is more appropriate than radio-therapy or stent placement due to speed of response.
- **Spinal cord compression:**
  - Both SCLC and NSCLC can metastasise to spinal vertebrae and progress to cause spinal cord compression.
  - Compression of the spinal cord causes a variety of signs and symptoms below the level of the lesion:
    - Back pain.
    - Numbness or paraesthesia.
    - Weakness or paralysis.
    - Hyperreflexia in presence of higher cord compression.
    - Loss of sensation.
    - Muscle weakness and wasting (chronic).
    - Bladder and bowel dysfunction.
    - Spinal shock: areflexia and motor paralysis.
    - Neurogenic shock: hypotension and bradycardia (cervical or thoracic lesion).
  - The gold standard test for suspected compression is spinal MRI.
    - CT myelography can be performed by experienced neuroradiolo-gists if MRI is not suitable e.g. in patients with older models of pacemakers.

- Spinal cord compression is a neuro-surgical emergency; diagnosis and treatment should not be delayed.
  - NICE guidelines state that treatment should be initiated within 24 hours of initial presentation.
- Treatment of compression due to malignancy includes:
  - Immobilisation, decompression and stabilisation surgery.
  - Corticosteroids (dexamethasone).
  - Radiotherapy.

MICRO-facts

If spinal cord compression is suspected in a patient, a thorough lower limb neurological exam and a per rectal (PR) exam MUST BE DONE. A PR exam is a sensitive test for demonstrating saddle anaesthesia and loss of anal tone, both of which are highly suggestive of spinal cord compression; they are signs of cauda equina syndrome.

Cauda equina syndrome:

Is caused by compression of the nerve roots caudal to the level of the spinal cord.

It is important as this type of compression usually progresses within hours or days.

Usually characterised by:

Saddle and perineal anaesthesia.

Bladder and bowel dysfunction (urinary retention and loss of anal tone).

Lower limb weakness and sensory deficit.

Lower back pain.

---

11. PROGNOSIS

- The prognosis of lung cancer varies depending on:
  - Type (e.g. SCLC or NSCLC)
  - Staging
  - Histological grading
  - Performance status
  - Treatment regimen and response.
- Survival rates are measured as the number of patients alive for 5 years or longer, after their initial cancer was diagnosed.
- Tables 5.4 and 5.5 show prognosis by cancer stage with treatment.

Respiratory Medicine

Table 5.4 **Prognosis of NSCLC with treatment, relative to the stage of the disease.**

STAGING OF NSCLC	5 YEAR SURVIVAL RATE
Stage IA1	92%
Stage 1A2	83%
Stage 1A3	77%
Stage IB	68%
Stage IIA	60%
Stage IIB	53%
Stage IIIA	36%
Stage IIIB	26%
Stage IIIC	13%
Stage IVA	10%
Stage IVB	0%

- If NSCLC recurs, prognosis is dependent on stage of the initial disease as well as stage of the recurrent cancer.
- SCLC has a worse prognosis, with the majority of patients dying within 2 years of diagnosis.

Table 5.5 **Prognosis of SCLC with treatment, relative to the stage of the disease.**

STAGING OF SCLC	5 YEAR SURVIVAL RATE
Limited	14–20%
Extensive	1–5%

- Recurrence of SCLC is almost universally fatal, median survival being 2–3 months.

MICRO-case
A patient with COPD presents with a suspected exacerbation. He has recently successfully quitted smoking. He has had a cough, which has persisted for the last 3 weeks, despite taking his prophylactic steroids and a course of antibiotics. His condition is stable and he denies increased breathlessness. A further course of antibiotics is prescribed and he is not sent to hospital. Two weeks later the cough still persists and the patient mentions that his sputum has become blood-flecked; on further questioning he has also recently lost some weight.   *continued...*

Respiratory Medicine

continued... The GP sends him for a chest X-ray which shows an opaque coin-like lesion in the right upper lobe and hilar lymphadenopathy. He is referred to chest clinic, on a 2-week wait. A bronchoscopy and biopsy of the mass confirms a diagnosis of small cell lung cancer. A staging CT shows that the disease is extensive involving other structures within the thorax. Chemotherapy and radiotherapy are started and prophylactic cranial irradiation planned. However, at his next appointment his gait is noted to be abnormal and he complains of recurrent headaches. A head CT demonstrates cerebral metastases.

Despite multiple rounds of treatment his condition steadily deteriorates. He begins to complain of weakness, nausea and vomiting. He also seems to be increasingly confused. Initially this was thought to be due to his cerebral metastases; however when blood tests are done he has hypercalcaemia. He is given 6 L of 0.9% saline, furosemide, zoledronic acid and gallium nitrate, and there is improvement. Despite this, it is decided at his next multi-disciplinary team (MDT) meeting that palliation should become the main aim of his care. He admits to struggling at home and so a joint decision is made to apply for hospice care. He is accepted to a hospice, where his general deterioration continues and he dies 3 weeks later, 9 months after his initial diagnosis.

Key Points

- A high index of suspicion for lung cancer is needed, especially in patients with concurrent lung disease.
- Delayed diagnosis can adversely affect prognosis.
- A biopsy with histological evidence of cancer is vital for diagnosis and planning for non-surgical disease modifying therapies.
- SCLC metastasises early; distant metastases can often be present at the time of diagnosis.
- SCLC has a poor prognosis than other types of primary lung cancer, especially if it is extensive. Treatment with curative intent may not be a viable option.
- The palliative care team should be involved early and the patient kept comfortable and symptom free, as far as is possible.

5.2 MESOTHELIOMA

. DEFINITION

- A malignant neoplasm arising from the epithelial cells that form the pleural lining of the lung.
  - Can also involve the peritoneum, pericardium or testis, however this is very rare.
- Subtypes include epithelioid (most common, better prognosis), sarcomatoid (worst prognosis) and biphasic (intermediate features of both).

2. EPIDEMIOLOGY

- Mesothelioma is more common in white ethnicity and males.
- It typically occurs in the older population, aged 50–80.
- The incidence has rapidly increased since the 1960s. The projected annual number of deaths was expected to peak in the UK around 2015 and then taper off. However, numbers have remained relatively stable.

3. AETIOLOGY

- Main risk factor for developing mesothelioma is asbestos exposure.
  - 80 – 90% of patients have a history of asbestos exposure.
- Latency between exposure and malignancy is 20 – 40 years.
- Smoking is associated with an increased risk of malignancy after exposure and it is known to worsen outcomes.
- Epidemiological studies and case reports suggest that exposure to radiation is associated with the development of mesothelioma.

MICRO-print

There are six types of asbestos identified, and they are divided into two groups (serpentine and amphibole):

Serpentine:
Chrysolite (most commonly used in buildings).

Amphibole:
Amosite
Crocidolite
Anthophyllite
Tremolite
Actinolite.

The most frequently used are also commonly categorised by their colour (tremolite, anthophyllite and actinolite are not classified in this system):

White asbestos: chrysolite
Brown asbestos: amosite
Blue asbestos: crocidolite.

Crocidolite (blue) asbestos is considered to be the most carcinogenic, with up to 18% of those exposed to it developing mesothelioma. This along with amosite (brown) asbestos has been banned in the UK since 1985. The sale and second hand re-use of chrysolite (white) asbestos became illegal in 1999.

Exposure to **ANY** type of asbestos is detrimental to health and has carcinogenic potential.

---

4. PRESENTATION

- The clinical features of mesothelioma are summarised in Figure 5.8.

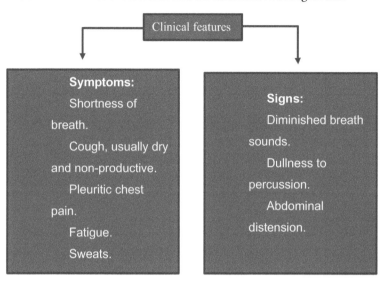

Figure 5.8 Clinical features of mesothelioma.

5. INVESTIGATION

- The investigation findings in mesothelioma are summarised in Table 5.6.

Table 5.6 **Investigations for a patient with suspected mesothelioma.**

INVESTIGATION	FINDINGS
Chest X-ray	Unilateral pleural effusion, irregular pulmonary fibrosis, reduced lung volume and parenchymal changes may be seen.
Chest CT	Pleural thickening, discrete pleural plaques, pleural and/or pericardial effusion, enlarge hilar and mediastinal lymph nodes and chest wall invasion may be seen.
Thoracentesis	Exudate may show malignant cells, however sensitivity of this test is relatively low.
Pleural biopsy	This is used to gain specimens for a definitive pathological diagnosis. It is usually CT guided or done during VATS.

Respiratory Medicine

6. MANAGEMENT

- Mesothelioma is considered incurable. Curative-intent multi-modality treatment is no longer carried out as the results of clinical trials did not demonstrate a clear benefit and was associated with significant treatment-related harm.
- Treatment decisions should be made through a specialist mesothelioma MDT (usually regional based).
- Some patients may be offered palliative surgery (extra-pleural decortication). The results of a UK-based clinical trial of this form of treatment are awaited.
- Fitter patients may be offered SACT (chemotherapy or immunotherapy), or may be entered into clinical trial.
- For malignant effusions, drainage, and talc pleurodesis can be effective. Performed by thoracoscopy or instillation of talc slurry via a closed chest tube.
    - A long term in-dwelling pleural catheter can be inserted if repeated drainage of a pleural infusion is needed (see Chapter 6)
- **Palliative care and symptomatic relief:**
    - Opiates, home oxygen and anxiolytics can have a role in parallel to other palliative and symptomatic control measures described above.

7. PROGNOSIS

- This is a highly lethal malignancy-median survival is 10 − 15 months.
    - Only 5 − 10% of patients survive to 5 years.
- Outlook is better in patients without mediastinal involvement and with epithelioid histology.

5.3 SECONDARY SPREAD OF SYSTEMIC MALIGNANCY TO LUNG AND PLEURA

1. AETIOLOGY

- Metastases to the lung from distant sites are common; most cancers have the ability to spread to the lung.
- The usual sites for the primary tumour are:
    - Kidney
    - Prostate
    - Bone
    - Breast
    - Gastrointestinal (GI) tract
    - Cervix
    - Ovary
    - Thyroid.

- Metastases usually occur in the parenchyma of the lung and can be relatively asymptomatic even with extensive disease.
- Lymphangitis carcinomatosa:
  - An inflammation of the lymphatics secondary to malignancy which can cause progressive breathlessness.
  - Lymphangitis carcinomatosa is usually due to secondary spread from stomach, pancreas or breast.

2. MANAGEMENT

- Treatment options taken are dependent on the site, type and extent of the primary tumour as well as the extent of the lung secondary.
  - If the secondary is an isolated early metastases, surgical intervention with curative intent can sometimes be performed.
  - Choice of chemotherapy, hormonal therapy or novel drugs depends on the histology and site of the primary tumour.

5.4 MEDIASTINAL MASSES

1. LYMPHOMA

- Can either represent disease isolated to mediastinum or as part of a more diffuse disease process:
  - Hodgkin's lymphoma.
  - Diffuse large B-cell lymphoma.
  - Lymphoblastic leukaemia/lymphocytic lymphoma.
  - Mucosal-associated lymphoid tissue (MALT) lymphoma.
- 50% of patients with disease limited to the thorax will be symptomless.

2. THYMOMA

- A primary pulmonary thymoma is a tumour originating from thymic tissue that presents in the lung of a patient with a normal thymus gland.
- Usually asymptomatic and often discovered as an incidental radiological anomaly.
- Patients may present with symptoms of myasthenia gravis and all should be screened for this.
- Relatively rare, they have no distinctive radiological features and immunohistochemistry studies are used for diagnosis.
- Surgical resection is usually curative unless the tumour is very extensive.
- Prognosis can be very good and is dependent upon complete resection and presence of local invasion.
- Post thymectomy, patients seem to be at increased risk of developing separate cancers, most commonly colorectal cancer.

Respiratory Medicine

3. EXTRAGONADAL GERM CELL TUMOURS (GCT)

- Mediastinal tumour of germ cell origin.
- There is an absence of primary disease within the testes or ovaries.
- Tumours are present in the midline and can be distributed in the following regions:
  - Retroperitoneum
  - Anterior mediastinal space
  - Pineal gland
  - Suprasellar cistern.
- Benign mature teratomas are the most common mediastinal GCT (> 50%) and tend to occur in adolescents.
  - Though benign, surgical excision is offered as they can transform to aggressive sarcomas and carcinomas.
- Seminomas are the most common malignant GCT and occur mainly in males.
  - Associated with elevated serum beta human chorionic gonadotrophin (bHCG) but not alpha fetoprotein (AFP).
  - Often has spread to lymph nodes and distant sites at presentation.
  - Usually very responsive to chemotherapy (>90% 5-year survival without extra-pulmonary distal metastases).
  - Malignant non-seminomatous GCTs include choriocarcinoma, egg yolk tumour and embryonal carcinoma.
  - They are likely to secrete serum (AFP).
  - Treatment is often multimodality with prognosis at 5 years being poor compared to seminomas.

4. OTHER MEDIASTINAL MASSES

- Thymic cancer.
- Retrosternal extension of thyroid mass.
- Cystic masses including:
  - Bronchogenic
  - Upper gastrointestinal
  - Pericardial.
- Neurogenic tumours:
  - Schwannomas
  - Ganglioneuromas.

Respiratory Medicine

Pleural Disease

6.1 PNEUMOTHORAX

1. DEFINITION

- A pneumothorax is an accumulation of air in the pleural space.
    - **Primary spontaneous pneumothorax (PSP):** A pneumothorax occurring in the presence apparently normal lungs.
    - **Secondary spontaneous pneumothorax (SSP):** A pneumothorax occurring in the presence of pre-existing underlying lung disease.
- **Tension pneumothorax:** Occurs when air is drawn in to the pleural space on inspiration but has no means of escape on expiration.
    - The increase in volume pushes the mediastinum into the contralateral hemithorax.
    - This leads to circulatory collapse and potential cardiorespiratory arrest.

2. EPIDEMIOLOGY

- Hospital admission rates for both PSP and SSP combined:
    - Men: 16.7/100000.
    - Women: 5.8/100000.
- Mortality rates:
    - Men: 1.26/*million*.
    - Women: 0.62/*million*.

> **MICRO-references**
> Gupta et al. Epidemiology of pneumothorax in England. *Thorax* 2000;
> 55 (8): 666–671

3. AETIOLOGY AND RISK FACTORS

- **Primary**:
    - Smoking tobacco and other illicit drugs (e.g. cannabis).
    - Tall, thin young males.

DOI: 10.1201/9781315113937-7

- Inherited disorders of collagen e.g. Marfan's syndrome.
- Some cases of PSP will be found to have evidence of small apical bullae if investigated with CT scan, even if no definite underlying lung disease is present.

- **Secondary:**
  - Often occurs due to rupture of emphysematous bullae in COPD.
  - Cystic lung disease e.g. Langerhans cell histiocytosis, pulmonary lymphangioleiomyomatosis (LAM).
  - Cystic fibrosis.
  - *Pneumocystis jirovecii* pneumonia.
- **Traumatic:**
  - Follows penetrating chest trauma.
- **Iatrogenic:**
  - Mechanical ventilation
  - Cardiac pacemaker implantation
  - Central line placement
  - Lung biopsy.
- **Female gender:**
  - Pulmonary ectopic endometriosis can cause rupture of a pleural bleb at time of menstruation (catamenial pneumothorax).
  - LAM is a rare condition characterised by abnormal smooth muscle proliferation leading to pneumothoraces and chylous effusions.

4. PATHOPHYSIOLOGY

- A communication is formed between an alveolus and the pleural space, or between the atmosphere and the pleural space.
  - This could be due to the rupture of a "bleb" or a penetrating chest injury.
- Gases flow along a pressure gradient into the pleural space.
  - Alveolar pressure > intrapleural pressure.
  - Atmospheric pressure > intrapleural pressure.
- This flow continues until the pressure gradient no longer exists or the communication is sealed.
- As a result of the accumulation of air in the pleural space, the lung reduces in volume.

5. CLINICAL FEATURES

- **Symptoms:**
  - Sudden onset chest pain (often pleuritic).
  - Shortness of breath.
- **Signs:**
  - Tachycardia.
  - If the pneumothorax is large enough:
    - Reduced chest expansion.
    - Hyper-resonant upon percussion of the affected side.
    - Quiet breath sounds on auscultation.
  - **Hamman's sign:** "Click" on auscultation in time with heart sounds. Occurs in left sided pneumothorax.
  - **Tension pneumothorax:**
    - Deviation of the trachea towards contralateral hemithorax.
    - Displaced apex beat.
    - **Pulsus paradoxus:** accentuated fall of systolic blood pressure with inspiration.
    - **In latter stages:** signs of poor cardiac output due to reduced venous return.

6. INVESTIGATIONS

- **Chest X-ray (CXR)**
  - Diagnostic in most cases, but look carefully around the periphery of the lung; always check the contralateral side because bilateral pneumothorax can occur (see Figures 6.1 and 6.2).
  - **Features:**
    - Visible lung edge against absent peripheral lung markings (See Figure 6.1).
    - May be difficult to visualise on supine films.
    - To measure size, estimate the horizontal distance between lung edge and chest wall at level of hilum.
    - A common mistake is to spot a "hilar mass" which is the completely collapsed lung.

Respiratory Medicine

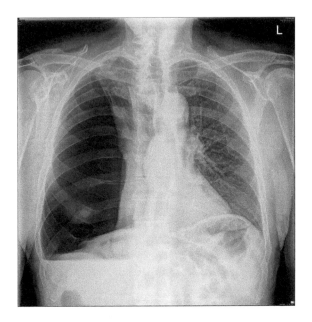

Figure 6.1 CXR of patient with a pneumothorax; the right lung field is radiolucent with visible lung marking near the right heart border and no lung markings peripherally to thi

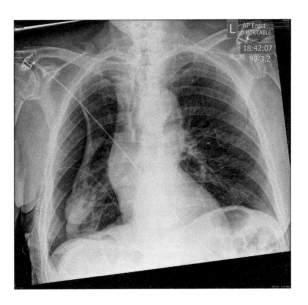

Figure 6.2 CXR of patient with pneumothorax; the right lung is partially collapsed an a chest drain has been inserted to treat the pneumothorax.

- **Tension pneumothorax:**
  - Deviation of trachea and mediastinum to the contralateral side.
    - ○ N.B. under normal circumstances a CXR should NEVER be performed if a tension pneumothorax is suspected, as this is a respiratory emergency.
- **Ultrasound** can detect even small pneumothoraces in skilled and experienced hands.
- **Arterial blood gas (ABG)**
  - Hypoxia.
  - Hypercapnia: may be present in secondary pneumothorax if it triggers decompensation of the pre-existing lung disease or in the late stages of tension pneumothorax development.
- **Computed tomography (CT) thorax**
  - Can be used to differentiate pneumothorax from bullous disease.
  - Use to search for underlying lung disease.

DIFFERENTIAL DIAGNOSIS (OF PRESENTING SYMPTOMS)

- Pleural effusion.
- Pulmonary embolus.
- Pleuritic chest pain from other causes e.g. pneumonia.

MANAGEMENT

- Depends on the presence or absence of symptoms, patient preference, whether the pneumothorax is of sufficient size to intervene safely, and whether it is primary or secondary.

Respiratory Medicine

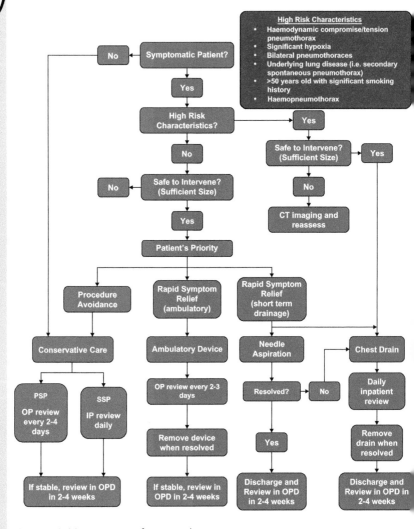

Figure 6.3 Management of pneumothorax.

MICRO-references
Flowcharts adapted from the British Thoracic Society Pleural Disease Guidelines 2023, available at:
    https://www.brit-thoracic.org.uk/quality-improvement/guidelines/pleural-disease/

- The British Thoracic Society has produced guidelines, updated in 2023. These are shown in Figure 6.3.
- For individuals with persistent air leak at 3–5 days, consider referral for definitive closure of air leak.
- Surgical management of spontaneous pneumothorax is usually undertaken via VATS and might include bullectomy, wedge excision of the part of the lung causing the air leak, as well as pleurectomy/pleural abrasion and talc insufflation to affect a permanent pleurodesis.
- Elective surgical management may be considered for a first episode of pneumothorax if in a high-risk occupation (e.g. airline pilot) or for tension pneumothorax at the first episode.
- Elective surgical management may also be considered for patients with a second ipsilateral or first contralateral pneumothorax.
- **Pleurodesis:**
  - Introduction of chemicals into the pleural space, used in the treatment of recurrent pneumothoraces.
  - Chemicals used include talc (most common), bleomycin, tetracycline and povidone iodine. A patient's own blood can also be used ("blood patch").
  - **For pneumothorax, chemical pleurodesis is usually reserved for individuals not suitable for surgery.**
- **Consider definitive surgical management in individuals presenting with a second pneumothorax.**
- For the management of tension pneumothorax, see Chapter 16: Respiratory Emergencies.

MICRO-facts

Chest Drain Indications and Insertion
Indications:
- Pneumothorax in a ventilated patient.
- Tension pneumothorax.
- PSP not resolving with needle aspiration.

continued...

Respiratory Medicine

continued...

- Large SSP.
- Malignant pleural effusion (see flowchart, below).
- Empyema/complicated parapneumonic effusion.
- Traumatic haemopneumothorax.
- Post operative.

Insertion:

- Informed consent must be gained and recorded.
- Aseptic technique should be used.
- Local anaesthetic infiltration is required.
- The chest tube should usually be inserted into the "safe triangle", which is bordered by:
  - Anterior border of latissimus dorsi.
  - Lateral border of pectoralis major.
  - A line superior to the horizontal level of the nipple.
  - An apex below the axilla.
- A Seldinger technique is used to insert the tube.
- The tube is secured with a suture.
- If possible insertion of a chest drain under ultrasound guidance is best practice.

MICRO-facts

Chest Drain Management and Removal

Management of the drainage system:

- The drain is usually attached to a closed underwater seal bottle, where the tube is underwater with a side vent to allow the escape of air. This allows only one direction of flow.
- The level of fluid in the tube should change with respiration. This is called "swing". Fluid levels should rise with inspiration and fall with expiration. Absence of swing suggests an occlusion or a misplaced tube (but can also occur when the lung is fully inflated).
- Bubbling in the underwater seal chamber suggests a continuing air leak but might also be a sign of a faulty connection or air entrained through the skin incision.
- In pleural effusion: drainage of >1.5 L in a short period can result in re-expansion pulmonary oedema and should be avoided.
- The drain site should be checked regularly for signs of infection.
- Suction may be used under some circumstances, e.g. in non-resolving pneumothorax.

continued...

continued...

Removing a chest drain:
> In pneumothorax, the chest drain should be removed when:

- There is confirmation of inflation of the lung on CXR with cessation of the air leak.
- There is cessation of any suction applied for >24 hours.
- There is cessation of bubbling in the underwater seal tube for >24 hours.

In pleural effusion/empyema, the chest drain should be removed when:

- Any sepsis has resolved.
- The output is low/dry.

The chest drain should be removed under aseptic technique, and is usually removed on expiration with the Valsalva manoeuvre (but don't worry too much about that). The drain site should be covered with a steristrip and the dressing applied. A suture may be needed for larger wounds and drains.

9. COMPLICATIONS

- **Complications of pneumothorax:**
  - Tension pneumothorax.
  - Sputum retention/infection.
  - Respiratory failure.
  - Circulatory failure.
  - Surgical emphysema – air tracks into the subcutaneous tissues causing swelling and a "crackling" sensation on palpation of the skin. Usually occurs after a drain has been inserted and implies that there is resistance to airflow through the drain, so check it is not blocked or kinked. If surgical emphysema is severe or progressing a new/larger drain may need to be placed. Seek senior advice.
- **Complications of treatment:**
  - **Re-expansion pulmonary oedema**
    - Follows evacuation of air from pleural space and rapid re-expansion of the collapse lung.
    - May occur if pneumothorax large and has been present for >72 hours.
    - Treatment is generally supportive.
  - **Talc pleurodesis-related ARDS (adult respiratory distress syndrome)**
    - Due to a systemic inflammatory response to the talc.

Respiratory Medicine

10. PROGNOSIS

- Complete resolution takes around 10 days in uncomplicated cases.
- Recurrence is common.
  - Ipsilateral recurrence can occur up to 49% at 1 year.
  - Contralateral recurrence can occur in 10%.
  - The probability of recurrence is higher if the patient:
    – Is >60 years old
    – Has pulmonary fibrosis
    – Has low weight for height
    – Continues to smoke.
  - The risk of fatality is higher in COPD (5%) and AIDS (25%).

MICRO-case

You are working as an ED SHO and are called to see a 68-year-old patient with COPD. He has presented with an acute worsening shortness of breath associated with a sharp stabbing chest pain, worse on inspiration. On examination he has a tachycardia, reduced chest expansion, hyper-resonance to percussion on the left side, associated with quiet breath sounds. You perform an ABG which shows:

$$pH : 7.28 \quad PaO_2 : 8 \ kPa \quad PaCO_2 : 7 \ kPa \quad HCO_3^- : 24 \ mmol/L$$

Chest radiograph reveals a visible rim of 1.5 cm between the lung margin and chest wall. As he is acutely breathless, requires inpatient care, and his priority is rapid symptomatic relief, you decide to aspirate with a 16G cannula. However, this is unsuccessful, with a rim >1 cm persisting on CXR. Consequently, you seek expert senior input to guide chest drain insertion and admit the patient to the respiratory ward.

Key Points

- The CXR can be used to quantify the size of a pneumothorax but size does not always correlate with clinical severity.
- Typically, SSP will have more physiological impact on the patient than PSP.
- Non-invasive ventilation is contraindicated to resolve type 2 respiratory failure until a chest drain is placed as positive pressure will worsen pneumothorax size.

6.2 PLEURAL EFFUSION

1. DEFINITION

- A small amount of pleural fluid is normally present with a close balance of production and reabsorption.

Respiratory Medicine

- A pleural effusion is an accumulation of fluid within the pleural space.
- They are usually defined as **transudative** or **exudative** (causes of each are listed in Table 6.1).

2. AETIOLOGY AND RISK FACTORS

- **Transudate:**
    - Imbalance of hydrostatic forces influencing pleural fluid formation and absorption, resulting in accumulation of pleural fluid.
- **Exudate:**
    - Increase in capillary/pleural surface permeability, resulting in fluid leakage, coupled with a reduced ability to reabsorb the generated fluid.

Table 6.1 **Causes of pleural effusion.**

	TRANSUDATIVE EFFUSIONS	EXUDATIVE EFFUSIONS
Common causes	Left ventricular failure	Malignancy
	Liver cirrhosis (usually with associated ascites)	Parapneumonic effusion (see MICRO-Facts box)
	Hypoalbuminaemia	Tuberculosis
	Peritoneal dialysis	Connective tissue disease
	Nephrotic syndrome	Pancreatitis
	Hypothyroidism	Asbestos (mesothelioma and benign asbestos pleural effusion)
	Mitral stenosis	Drugs e.g. methotrexate
Rare causes	Meigs syndrome (right sided effusion secondary to ovarian fibroma)	Post-myocardial infarction
	Superior vena cava obstruction	Sarcoidosis
	Constrictive pericarditis	Yellow nail syndrome (secondary to lymphedema)
	Ovarian hyperstimulation.	Familial Mediterranean fever
	Malignancy (most are exudates)	

> ## MICRO-facts
>
> **Parapneumonic Effusions**
>
> - Uncomplicated: resolves with antibiotic therapy alone.
> - Complicated: requires pleural space drainage (defined as pH < 7.2) and treated as if empyema.
> - Empyema (presence of pus macroscopically or positive bacterial culture): end stage parapneumonic effusion. (See Chapter 2: Respiratory infections.)

3. PATHOPHYSIOLOGY

- Pleural effusions arise as an imbalance of the production and removal of the fluid in the pleural space.
  - Fluid enters the potential space from the capillaries of the parietal pleura.
  - It is removed by the lymphatics of the parietal pleura.
- Under normal circumstances, a small amount of fluid is necessary to lubricate the cavity and allow movement of the lung within the thorax.
  - Approximately 20 mL per hemithorax.
- Disruption of fluid balance can be a result of local or systemic derangements:
  - **Local changes** including infection, trauma or infarction cause increased permeability of the capillaries. Malignant disease and inflammation can impair the ability of lymphatics to remove the generated fluid.
    - The fluid is called an **exudate** and is protein and LDH rich.
  - **Systemic changes** include decreased oncotic pressure, increased capillary pressure and the presence of ascites.
    - These cause net movement of fluid out of the capillaries; permeability is not altered.
    - The fluid is called a **transudate** and has a low protein and LDH content.

4. CLINICAL FEATURES

- Symptoms:
  - Effusions can be asymptomatic in individuals who have a relatively normal contralateral lung.
  - Shortness of breath.
  - Cough.
  - Chest pain.

- Important features in the history:
  - Features suggestive of malignancy:
    - Loss of weight
    - Persistent chest pain
    - Smoking history
    - Asbestos exposure.
- Signs:
  - Reduced chest expansion on the ipsilateral side.
  - Deviation of the trachea away from the affected side with large pleural effusions.
    - Deviation may be towards the affected side if there is a lung collapse.
  - Dullness to percussion.
  - Diminished breath sounds.
  - Loss of vocal resonance.

MICRO-facts

Classical CXR Appearance

- Concave upper border reflecting fluid meniscus.
- Mediastinal deviation: away from affected side with large effusions.
- Drawing of the trachea to the affected side may reflect underlying collapse due to an obstructing mass.

---

5. INVESTIGATIONS

- **Chest X-ray:**
  - Approximately 200 mL of fluid has accumulated when there is visible loss of the costophrenic angle on a posterior-anterior (PA) CXR (see Figure 6.4).

Respiratory Medicine

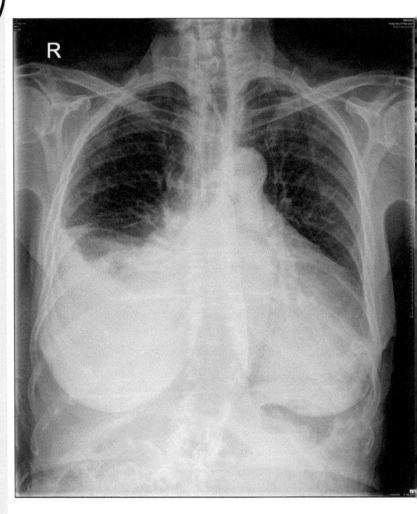

Figure 6.4 CXR of a patient with bilateral pleural effusion; there is loss of costophrenic angles at both sides, with opacity in the lower lung fields on both sides. A fluid meniscus can be seen in the right lung.

- **Blood tests to identify underlying cause:**
  - FBC/CRP (may suggest infection).
  - LFTs.
  - Serum LDH.
  - Serum glucose.
  - TFTs.
  - Ensure clotting studies are done if aspiration required.
  - Tumour markers if a specific malignancy suspected.
- **Ultrasound:**
  - Ultrasound is more sensitive than CXR, and is able to detect even small pleural effusions.
  - Drainage or diagnostic aspiration of a pleural effusion should be done under ultrasound guidance.
- **Diagnostic aspiration:**
  - Send sample for pH and specific biochemical, cytological and microbiological tests.
  - The appearance of the aspirated fluid may give an indication of the cause of the effusion (see Table 6.2).

Table 6.2 **Appearance of pleural fluid and likely causes.**

APPEARANCE	POSSIBLE CAUSE
Bloody	Trauma, malignancy, pulmonary infarction, pneumonia, post-cardiac injury, pneumothorax, asbestos-related, aortic dissection or rupture.
Turbid/milky	Empyema, chylothorax or pseudochylothorax.
Putrid odour	Anaerobic empyema.
Food particles	Oesophageal rupture (Boerhaave's syndrome).
Urine odour	Urinothorax (occurs rarely secondary to obstructive uropathy).
Black	Aspergillus infection.
Brown "anchovy sauce"	Amoebic liver abscess draining in to pleural space.

- **Biochemistry**
  - Protein.
    - **Transudate:** pleural fluid protein <30 g/L.
    - **Exudate:** pleural fluid protein >30 g/L.
    - In borderline cases use **Light's Criteria** (see MICRO-Facts box).
  - LDH.

Respiratory Medicine

- **Cytology**
  - Increased neutrophil count suggests empyema.
  - Increased lymphocyte count is very common in a variety of scenarios but may suggest TB, connective tissue disorders or lymphoproliferative disorders.
  - Increased red cell number occurs in malignancy, trauma, haemothorax and PE.
  - Pleural fluid should be routinely assessed for malignant cells.
- **Microbiology**
  - Gram stain, MC&S.
  - AFB stain and culture.
- **pH**
  - Measure in arterial blood gas syringe within 1 hour of aspiration to ensure accuracy.
  - **pH < 7.2 should raise suspicion of empyema and need to perform drainage.**

MICRO-facts

Light's Criteria

Pleural fluid is exudative if ≥1 criteria are met:

- Pleural fluid protein divided by serum protein is >0.5.
- Pleural fluid LDH divided by serum LDH is >0.6.

Pleural fluid LDH is more than two-thirds the upper limits of normal serum LDH.

- **Biopsy of pleural tissue:** radiologically guided percutaneous needle biopsy is of particular value in diagnosing malignancy or tuberculosis (TB). Perform if:
  - Undiagnosed exudative effusion.
  - Non-diagnostic cytology.
  - Clinical suspicion of TB or malignancy.
  - Performed either by CT or by ultrasound scan (USS) technique.
- **Thoracoscopy:** an endoscopic technique used for visualisation of the lungs, pleura and mediastinum and collection of tissue samples.
  - Can be performed under light sedation or under general anaesthesia.
  - Allows evacuation of pleural fluid during procedure.
  - Deflation of the lung during the procedure (either by introduction of air via a three-way tap across the chest wall or clamping of the endotracheal tube ventilating the affected hemithorax) prevents re-expansion pulmonary oedema when pleural fluid is removed during thoracoscopy.

DIFFERENTIAL DIAGNOSIS

- Pleural thickening
- Pulmonary collapse/consolidation
- Elevated hemidiaphragm
- Pleural malignancy:
  - Secondary
  - Mesothelioma.

MANAGEMENT

- The management of pleural effusion according to updated BTS guidelines is summarised in Figures 6.5 and 6.6.

Observation:
- Often no intervention is necessary in small pleural effusions.

Pleural fluid tap:
- If the effusion is symptomatic, it can be drained using the same procedure as a diagnostic tap.
- Aspiration >1.5 L in one sitting can precipitate re-expansion pulmonary oedema and should therefore be avoided.

Chest drain insertion:
- Appropriate for active pleural infection, known malignancy and used cautiously for all effusions if there is respiratory failure.
- Aggressive drainage of transudative effusions can precipitate fluid shift and possible acute kidney injury (AKI).

Thoracoscopy (see above):
- Useful to provide both diagnosis and therapeutic management of exudative effusions.

Indwelling drainage:
- For recurrent effusions or when underlying lung tissue does not fully inflate ("trapped lung").
- A pleural catheter is inserted and tunnelled under the skin (similar to a Hickman line).
- This helps minimise infection risk in patients where long-term drainage is required.

Pleurodesis with talc:
- Primarily for malignant effusions.

Pleurectomy.

Pleuroperitoneal shunt:
- Used when the above measures are unsuccessful.

Respiratory Medicine

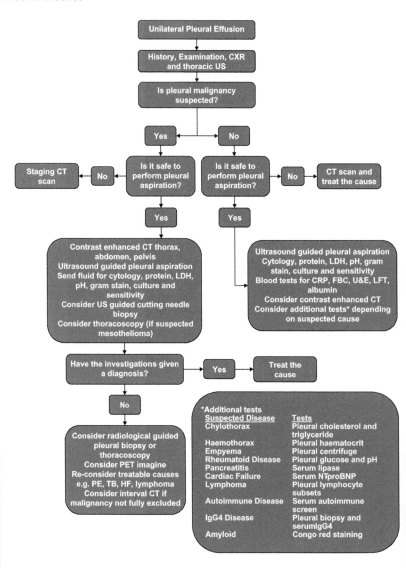

Figure 6.5 Investigation and management of unilateral pleural effusion.

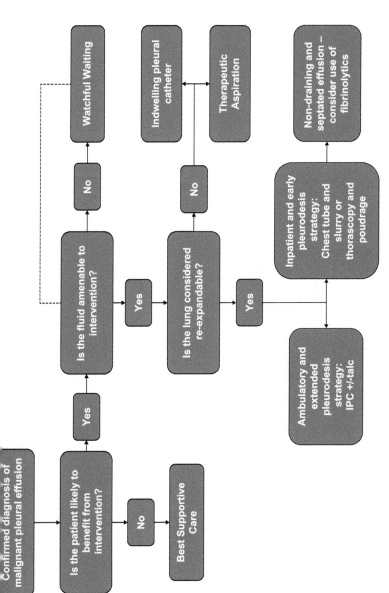

Figure 6.6

Respiratory Medicine

8. COMPLICATIONS

- Complications may be a consequence of the primary pathology e.g. malignancy or heart failure.
- **Complications of effusion:**
  - Atelectasis.
  - Passive lobar collapse due to volume of fluid.
  - Pleural thickening and fibrosis.
  - Pseudochylothorax: cholesterol-rich effusion due to chronic pleural inflammation, usually >5 years.
  - Trapped lung secondary to visceral pleural thickening.
- **Complications of treatment:**
  - Pneumothorax secondary to thoracocentesis.
  - Re-expansion pulmonary oedema.

9. PROGNOSIS

- Prognosis is related to underlying cause.
  - Malignancy of the pleural cavity reflects incurable disease.

MICRO-case
You are a respiratory physician clerking a 70-year-old gentleman, Mr. Tyler, who has been referred by his GP with shortness of breath and pleuritic chest pain. On clinical examination he has a dull percussion note and reduced breath sounds on the left side. A pleural effusion is confirmed on CXR; however the aetiology is not clear based on the clinical history.

You arrange for pleural aspiration to be performed under ultrasound guidance and send the sample for analysis, requesting protein and LDH levels; microbiology; cytology and pH. In addition you send blood for serum protein and LDH levels.

The results show a protein level of 35 g/L. As this is close to the threshold of 30 g/L, you use Light's criteria to confirm that the fluid is exudative as the pleural protein: serum protein ratio is 0.6 and the pleural LDH: serum LDH ratio is 0.68. Cytology

continued...

continued...
of the aspirate reveals the presence of malignant cells. You suspect lung cancer on the basis of Mr. Tyler's smoking history of 50 pack-years which is confirmed on CT thorax.

As Mr Tyler is likely to benefit from intervention and the lung is considered re-expandable, you decide to drain the effusion and perform talc pleurodesis. This procedure is successful.

Key Points

- Light's criteria are used in borderline cases to determine whether an effusion is transudative or exudative.
- Malignancies are the main cause of exudative pleural effusions.
- The primary malignancies most commonly associated with pleural effusions include lung cancer, breast cancer and lymphoma.
- Management of malignant effusions is guided by prognosis and symptomatic improvement.

Respiratory Medicine

7 Pulmonary Embolism

1. DEFINITION

- Occlusion of the pulmonary vasculature, usually caused by a thrombus which arises from the deep veins of the pelvis or lower limb.
- Amniotic fluid, air embolism and fat embolism can also occur.

2. EPIDEMIOLOGY

- The risk of venous thromboembolism is $1-1.5$ per 1000 person-years, but varies widely depending on risk factors (see below)
- Other causes of pulmonary embolism are less common.

3. AETIOLOGY AND RISK FACTORS

- The risk factors for venous thromboembolism are:
  - Surgery: particularly major abdominal/pelvic or lower limb surgery or intensive care treatment post-operatively.
  - Pregnancy and puerperium.
  - Caesarean section.
  - Lower limb fracture.
  - Immobility.
  - Malignancy: particularly advanced disease or abdominal/pelvic cancer.
  - Trauma.
  - Hormone replacement therapy/oral contraceptive pill.
  - Thrombotic disorders.
    - Factor V Leiden, protein C and S deficiency, antithrombin deficiency.
  - Myeloproliferative disorders.
  - Nephrotic syndrome.
  - Long-distance sedentary travel.

4. PATHOPHYSIOLOGY

- Effects of the pulmonary embolism are determined by the amount of pulmonary circulation that is affected.
  - **Massive pulmonary embolism:**

DOI: 10.1201/9781315113937-8

- PE with haemodynamic instability:
  - ○ Hypotension: SBP < 90 mmHg.
  - ○ Postural BP drop.
  - ○ Syncope.
- Associated significant thrombus load on CTPA causing right ventricular outflow obstruction, with radiological features of right heart strain
- **Hypoxaemia in massive PE occurs due to ventilation-perfusion mismatch:**
  - ○ Affected areas of the lung are ventilated but not perfused due to obstruction of pulmonary blood flow.
  - ○ Increased blood flow to unaffected areas of the lung can also occur.
  - ○ These alveoli are unable to sufficiently oxygenate the additional blood volume, resulting in low PaO2.

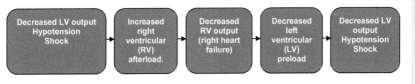

Figure 7.1 Pathophysiology of haemodynamic instability in massive PE.

- **Submassive pulmonary embolism:**
  - Significant thrombus load causing signs of right heart strain on imaging tests but with absence of cardiovascular compromise.

5. CLINICAL FEATURES

- Clinical features of PE and DVT are summarised in Table 7.1.

Table 7.1 **Clinical features of PE and DVT.**

SYMPTOMS OF PE	SIGNS OF PE	SIGNS OF DVT
Dyspnoea	Cyanosis	Leg swelling
Pleuritic chest pain	Tachycardia	Tenderness
Haemoptysis	Tachypnoea	Erythema
Dizziness	Hypotension/Postural BP drop	Warmth
Syncope	Raised JVP	Engorged superficial veins
	Pleural rub	
	Pleural effusion	
	Gallop rhythm	

Respiratory Medicine

7.1 CLINICAL MANAGEMENT OF PE

1. INVESTIGATIONS

- **Basic investigations**
  - A number of generic tests will be required if PE is suspected.
  - **CXR:** often normal and more helpful in excluding other diagnoses. Findings can only be suggestive, not diagnostic, of PE.
    - Atelectasis.
    - Fleischner's sign: prominent central pulmonary artery.
    - Westermark's sign: oligaemia in PE area of distribution (see Figure 7.1)
    - Small pleural effusion.
  - **ECG:** not diagnostic as an isolated test.
    - Sinus tachycardia.
    - New right axis deviation.
    - New right bundle branch block (See Figure 7.2).
    - Atrial fibrillation
    - $S_1Q_3T_3$ – S wave in lead I, with Q wave and inverted T wave in lead III.
  - **ABG:** hypoxia and hypocapnia are suggestive of PE.

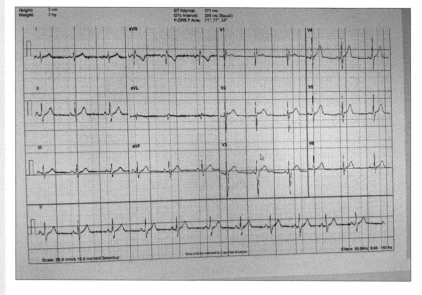

Figure 7.2 An ECG showing right bundle branch block.

- **Clinical risk scoring**
  - Any further investigations will be determined by the clinical judgement and clinical risk scoring.

Respiratory Medicine

- The most commonly used clinical risk scores are the Wells score (see Table 7.2) or the Geneva score (see Table 7.3).
- The Wells score is simpler and used more commonly in the UK.
  - Wells score:
    - >4 – high risk
    - ≤4 – a low risk (although 8% of low risk patients will have a PE).
  - Geneva Score:
    - ≤4 – low probability (10%)
    - 5–8 – intermediate probability (38%)
    - >8 – high probability (81%)
- The pre-test score determines choice of investigation (See Figure 7.4).

Table 7.2 **Wells Score for PE.**

CLINICAL FEATURE	SCORE
Clinical signs and symptoms of DVT.	Yes: +3
PE most, or equally most, likely possibility.	Yes: +3
Heart rate >100.	Yes: +1.5
Immobilisation for at least 3 days, or surgery in previous 4 weeks.	Yes: +1.5
Previous history of PE/DVT	Yes: +1.5
Haemoptysis	Yes: +1
Malignancy: palliative or with treatment in last 6 months.	Yes: +1

Table 7.3 **Geneva Score for PE.**

VARIABLE	CRITERIA	SCORE
Age	60–79 years	1
	>80 years	2
Past history PE/DVT		2
Surgery within last 4 weeks		3
Heart rate	>100 bpm	1
$PaCO_2$	<35 mmHg	2
	35–39 mmHg	1
PaO_2	<49 mmHg	4
	49–59 mmHg	3
	60–71 mmHg	2
	72–82 mmHg	1
Chest X-ray findings	Band atelectasis	1
	Elevated hemidiaphragm	1

Respiratory Medicine

- **Further Tests:**
  - If there is sufficient clinical suspicion or the clinical risk scoring indicates, further tests are required:
  - **D-dimer** has a 96% sensitivity, but low specificity.
    - Should not be used as a routine test but can be useful to exclude PE if there is a low-risk Wells score.
      - ○ A low-risk Wells score and negative D-dimer indicates a very low likelihood PE and usually is interpreted as excluding the diagnosis of PE.
      - ○ In other situations a negative D-dimer lacks negative predictive value and further tests are required to confirm or exclude.
  - Ventilation-perfusion nuclear medicine (VQ) scan
    - A gamma camera is used to record the distribution of inhaled and peripherally infused radio-labelled technetium. The images from the two phases are compared to look for unmatched defects in perfusion.
    - May be offered as an alternative to CTPA in certain patients:
      - ○ Allergy to contrast media
      - ○ Severe renal impairment
      - ○ High risk from irradiation
    - Does not provide additional diagnostic or prognostic information although can provide an estimation of clot burden.
  - CT pulmonary angiogram **(CTPA)** is a highly specific test for the diagnosis of a PE (See Figure 7.3):
    - This is the most commonly used diagnostic test.
    - The contrast agent may cause nephrotoxicity in patients with significant renal impairment.
    - Provides clear visual assessment of the clot burden, can show signs of right heart strain (for prognostication) and may provide an alternative diagnosis if PE is not seen.
    - More limited in ability to detect small subsegmental clots especially if breathing artefact or incorrect timing of contrast injection.
  - **Pulmonary angiography:** the gold standard for the diagnosis/exclusion of a PE.
    - It is invasive (right heart catheterisation) and has associated morbidity and mortality.
    - Rarely performed unless mechanical disruption or thrombectomy is anticipated.
  - **Transthoracic echo (TTE):** may be done in patients to identify right ventricular (RV) strain, but not often used acutely as RV strain can be recognised on CTPA.

Respiratory Medicine

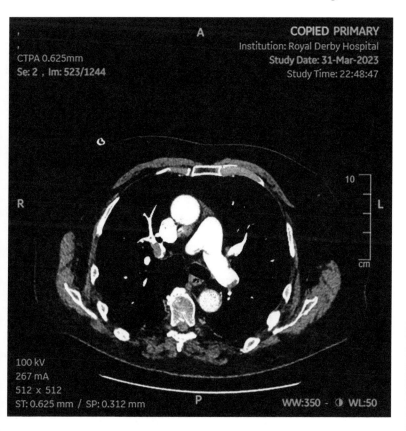

Figure 7.3 A CTPA scan in a patient with a central PE.

- – May occasionally identify a thrombus in the right heart.
- **Cardiac biomarkers:** used to predict prognostic course.
  - – **BNP/NT-proBNP:** increased levels reflect the severity of haemodynamic compromise.
  - – **Troponin T:** a marker of myocardial damage, associated with a poorer prognosis.
- **Investigations for malignancy** should be considered in all patients with unprovoked DVT/PE:
  - – Assessment should include:
    - ○ Review of medical history
    - ○ Baseline blood tests including FBC, U&E, liver function tests, and physical examination

Respiratory Medicine

- Routine abdominal/pelvic imaging is no longer recommended, but can be considered in those where there is suspicion of cancer from the above work-up.
- **Thrombophilia screen** can be considered in patients with unprovoked PE but should not be done if anticoagulation is expected to continue indefinitely.

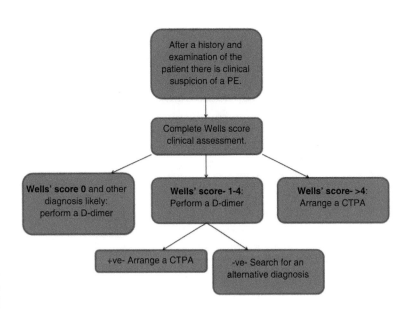

Figure 7.4 Suggested evaluation for PE based on Wells Score.

2. DIFFERENTIAL DIAGNOSIS

- Symptoms of PE are shared with other cardiac and respiratory conditions:
  - Angina.
  - Myocardial infarction.
  - Pericarditis.
  - Exacerbation of congestive heart failure.
  - Cardiac tamponade.
  - Pneumonia.
  - Acute exacerbation of COPD (chronic obstructive pulmonary disease).
  - Acute exacerbation of asthma.
  - Pneumothorax.
  - Dysfunctional breathing/anxiety disorders.

Respiratory Medicine

3. MANAGEMENT

- Treatment is dependent on the extent of the PE and the haemodynamic stability of the patient.
  - Initial management of the haemodynamically unstable patient is covered in Chapter 16: Respiratory emergencies.
- **Empirical anticoagulation** should begin without delay (unless contraindicated).
  - **Low molecular weight heparin (LMWH):** e.g. dalteparin, enoxaparin, tinzaparin.
    - LMWH is the treatment of choice.
    - Administered as a daily or twice daily subcutaneous injection.
    - The dose is calculated according to the patient's body weight.
    - Factor Xa monitoring may be required in patients at an increased risk of bleeding or at the extremes of body weight.
  - **Unfractionated heparin** is used in renal failure or patients where very quick reversal is needed (e.g. immediately post-operatively).
    - Give initial dose of 5000 units or 75 units/kg IV followed by 18 units/kg/hour.
    - Daily monitoring of APTT (activated partial thromboplastin time) is required.
  - Directly acting oral anticoagulant (DOAC) – may be used in the outpatient setting in low-risk patients.
- **Thrombolysis:** consider if the patient is haemodynamically compromised (SBP < 90 mmHg) or shocked (see Chapter 16: Respiratory Emergencies).
  - Systemic thrombolysis with alteplase is first choice for massive PE.
  - Catheter-directed thrombolysis may also be performed.
  - There is a 10% risk of a major bleed if thrombolysis is used.
- **Embolectomy:** consider if there is a high risk of bleeding or thrombolysis has failed.
  - Done surgically or by intrapulmonary arterial catheter.
- **Inferior vena cava (IVC) filter:**
  - Used if anticoagulation therapy is not appropriate and there is a lower limb venous thromboembolism.
  - Removal of the IVC should be considered once the patient is able to take anticoagulants.
- **Ongoing anticoagulation:**
  - After initial treatment, anticoagulation should continue for a minimum of 3 months.
  - 3 months of treatment is considered adequate in patients with a provoked PE, whereas lifelong treatment is often recommended in unprovoked PE depending on the balance of risks of recurrence and bleeding (see MICRO-Facts box).

Respiratory Medicine

- Options include continued LMWH, warfarin or a DOAC. DOACs have become the treatment of choice in the past couple of years due to efficacy and ease of use.
  - Always check for any drug interactions and caution is needed in renal impairment.
- Bridging LMWH can be stopped immediately if a DOAC is used, but if loading with warfarin should be continued until INR is $2.0 - 3.0$ for two consecutive days.

MICRO-references

In 2016 NICE released guidelines that include a framework for the diagnosis and treatment of VTE, available at:

www.nice.org.uk/guidance/ng158/chapter/Recommendations

In 2018 the British Thoracic Society released guidelines on the Outpatient management of Pulmonary Embolism, available at:

www.brit-thoracic.org.uk/document-library/guidelines/ambulatory-pe/bts-guideline-for-the-initial-outpatient-management-of-pulmonary-embolism/

---

4. COMPLICATIONS

- Complications from pulmonary embolism are either acute (during the initial event) or chronic (see Table 7.4).

Table 7.4 **Complications of PE.**

ACUTE	CHRONIC
Pulmonary infarction	Pulmonary hypertension
Cardiorespiratory arrest	Recurrent emboli
Due to treatment:	
Bleeding	Heparin-induced thrombocytopenia

MICRO-print

Heparin-Induced Thrombocytopenia

- Due to antibodies formed against complexes of platelet factor 4 and heparin.
- Usually occurs 5–14 days after commencing treatment with heparin.
- More common with use of UFH compared with LMWH.
- Typically presents with venous thrombosis rather than bleeding.
- Other clinical features:

continued…

Respiratory Medicine

continued...

- Venous limb gangrene.
- Skin lesions at injection sites.
- Systemic reactions to heparin boluses.
- Adrenal infarction.
- Arterial thrombosis.
- Platelet counts typically fall by >50% of their baseline value.
- If suspected, heparin should be discontinued.

5. PROGNOSIS

- Patient outcomes correlate with their clinical condition and haemodynamic stability at presentation:
  - Patients with SBP < 90 mmHg have a 31–58% mortality rate.
  - Patients with a SBP > 90 mmHg have a 3% mortality rate.
  - An elevated D-dimer is associated with increased mortality.

MICRO-case

A 37-year-old women, who is 7 months pregnant, presents to her GP with a 4-hour history of chest pain and shortness of breath. During the consultation the GP notes that she has also been suffering with leg pain over the last couple of days. On examination the GP notes that neither of her legs is red or swollen and her chest is clear. However, she complains of tenderness on palpation of her left calf. She is also tachypnoeic, with a respiration rate (RR) of 28.

The GP suspects a PE and calls an ambulance and she is transferred to A&E.

On arrival in A&E her respiration rate is now 35 and she is haemodynamically unstable with an SBP of 76. An ECG performed on arrival shows sinus tachycardia and signs of RV strain. She is started on high-flow O_2, fluid resuscitated and stabilised before being sent for a CTPA. Due to the high probability of a PE she is given a bolus of 5000 units of unfractionated heparin. She is also given a dose of steroids, due to the risk that she will labour prematurely.

Her CTPA scan shows a large PE. However, she is now stable and low-molecular-weight heparin (LMWH) is commenced. The patient makes a full recovery and is discharged from hospital. Her pregnancy continues to term and her LMWH is stopped 4 months after her delivery.

Respiratory Medicine

8 Tuberculosis

8.1 PULMONARY TUBERCULOSIS

1. DEFINITION

- Development of tuberculosis requires infection by one of the *Mycobacterium* tuberculosis complex organisms – *M. tuberculosis, M. bovis* or *M. africanum.*
- Tuberculosis (TB) is primarily a pulmonary infection; however it can disseminate to other organ systems.
- Active pulmonary TB implies inadequate containment by the immune system.
- Infections can be categorised as:
  - Primary (immediate disease onset post-infection).
  - Latent (asymptomatic infection).
  - Secondary/post-primary (reactivation of latent infection).
  - Extra-pulmonary/miliary.

2. EPIDEMIOLOGY

- UK 1.4 cases per 1,000 people.
- > 70% patients are born outside of UK.
- Other risk factors include:
  - Male sex.
  - Older age.
  - History of imprisonment.
  - Substance misuse.
  - Homelessness.
  - Chronic disease (such as diabetes, CKD, liver impairment).
  - Immunosuppression.
- More details available here: www.gov.uk/government/publications/ tuberculosis-in-england-2022-report-data-up-to-end-of-2021/ tb-incidence-and-epidemiology-in-england-2021

DOI: 10.1201/9781315113937-9

3. PATHOPHYSIOLOGY

- The majority of human TB infection is caused by *M. tuberculosis*.
  - Spread is via aerosol route.
- *M. bovis* is causative in areas with poor agricultural control measures and is spread directly from animals to farm workers or via unpasteurised milk.
- *M. africanum* is causative in West Africa but is less prevalent or pathogenic than *M. tuberculosis*.
- 5 – 10% patients with latent TB will develop reactivated TB.

4. CLINICAL FEATURES

- Clinical features of primary and secondary TB are summarised in table 8.1.

Table 8.1 **Comparison between primary and secondary TB.**

	PRIMARY TB	SECONDARY TB
Onset	Primary TB occurs within 12 months of transmission of the pathogen to a new host.	Secondary (post-primary) TB occurs 5 years or more after the primary infection, occurs in only 5% of those who are infected.
Symptoms	Febrile illness Cough Sputum production Haemoptysis Chest pain.	Night sweats Cough + mucoid or purulent sputum Haemoptysis Chest pain: pleuritic Weight loss: anorexia.
Signs	Chest: Bronchial breathing. ↓ Chest expansion. Dullness on percussion (effusion). Erythema nodosum. Phlyctenular conjunctivitis (inflammation of the conjunctivae along with the formation of small red nodules of lymphoid tissue). Lymphadenopathy.	Fever. Clubbing. Erythema nodosum. Respiratory signs: Apical crackles. Apical bronchial breathing. Wheeze. Signs consistent with pleural effusion.
Chest X-ray appearance	Ghon complex: central zone cavitation + hilar lymphade-nopathy (see Figure 8.1). Consolidation. Pleural effusion.	Apical consolidation and cavitation. Hilar lymphadenopathy (see Figure 8.1) Pleural effusion.

Respiratory Medicine

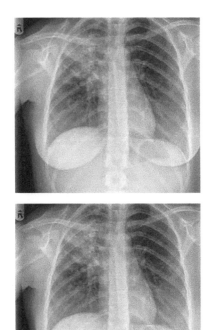

Figure 8.1 CXR of patient with TB; the image shows characteristic hilar lymphadenopathy and a cavitating lesion.

- Late and extra-pulmonary features: These are due to a direct progression of the infection to disseminated miliary (tertiary) TB.
  - Lobar collapse
  - Pericardial effusion
  - Meningitis
  - Osteomyelitis
  - Renal and skin disease.
- Extra-pulmonary/miliary TB: occurs with TB usually as a consequence of an initial pulmonary infection.

Respiratory Medicine

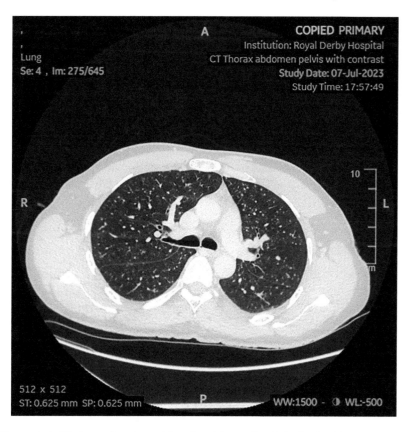

Figure 8.2 CT chest of patient with miliary TB; small, calcified millet-like lesions are seen throughout the lung.

MICRO-references

The Green Book is an up-to-date presentation of the current evidence and UK Department of Health (DoH) guidelines for population immunisation against infectious diseases including BCG vaccination:

www.gov.uk/government/collections/immunisation-against-infectious-disease-the-green-book

NICE guidelines covering prevention, identification and management of latent and active tuberculosis (TB) in children, young people and adults:

www.nice.org.uk/guidance/ng33

Respiratory Medicine

- Bacillaemia during the initial infection leads to mycobacterial complexes being deposited in multiple organ systems. (See section 8.2 for further details).

5. INVESTIGATIONS

- **Pulmonary tuberculosis can mimic many other respiratory conditions.** Tests would be done to rule out another cause of pneumonia (see Chapter 5.4).
- Tuberculin skin test (TST) (in UK, perform Mantoux as per the UK Department of Health (DoH) Green Book), or Interferon-Gamma Release Assay (IGRA) (see MicroFacts below). It is important to remember that a positive test implies infection rather than disease, but the IGRA is unaffected by prior BCG vaccination.

MICRO-facts

Tuberculin Skin Test

- Tuberculin is a purified protein derivative extracted from *Mycobacterium tuberculosis*.
- The tuberculin is injected subcutaneously on the lower part of the patient's arm.
- The patient returns within 48–72 hours and the induration in response to the injection is measured.
- A 15 mm induration is considered to be a positive test and evidence of current or past infection with TB. (NB. In higher risk groups an induration of 5 or 10 mm may be considered positive.)
  - Further testing is then needed to confirm the diagnosis.

Interferon-Gamma Release Assay

- A fresh blood sample is taken from a patient.
- The blood sample is mixed with M. tuberculosis antigens. If the patient has ever been infected with TB their white blood cells will react to the antigens by releasing interferon gamma.
- A positive test indicates past (latent) or current active infection with TB, but cannot differentiate.

- Chest X-ray:
  - Chest CT can be considered if there is diagnostic doubt.
- Every effort should be made to confirm the presence of the organism in a suitable specimen, such as:
  - Sputum (expectorated or induced using hypertonic saline).
  - Pleural sampling (higher yield with biopsy vs. fluid).
  - Bronchoalveolar lavage (BAL).

- Early morning urine sample for renal or miliary TB.
- Biopsy from an extra-pulmonary site.
- Using suitable specimens there are a number of methods used to identify the presence of acid fast bacilli (AFB):
  - Microscopic examination using:
    - Ziehl-Neelson stain.
    - Fluorescent staining: auramine or rhodamine B.
  - Culture on solid media:
    - Lowenstein-Jensen media (takes 8 weeks).
  - Liquid culture:
    - Mycobacterium growth indicator tube (MGIT) system (takes 3–14 days).
  - PCR (rapid with 100% sensitivity).
- All patients with confirmed TB should be tested for HIV.

6. DIFFERENTIAL DIAGNOSIS

- Community-acquired pneumonia
- Non-tuberculous *Mycobacterium*
- Lung cancer
- Sarcoidosis
- Wegner's granulomatosis
- Lymphoma.

7. COMPLICATIONS

- Immune reconstitution inflammatory syndrome (IRIS).
- Pneumothorax.
- Empyema.
- Parenchymal lung destruction/bronchiectasis.
- Catastrophic haemoptysis.

MICRO-print

Immune reconstitution inflammatory syndrome: a clinical phenomenon observed in patients recovering from immunodeficiency. An inflammatory flare occurs during rapid immune reconstitution targeted against an infective agent (viable or non-viable). It can occur in patients undergoing treatment for HIV/AIDS with concurrent or previously treated TB. Although most cases self-resolve, it can on occasion be an overwhelming and life-threatening reaction.

Respiratory Medicine

8. PROGNOSIS

- Mortality rate of > 50% in untreated patients.
- Fatalities rare with adequate treatment.
- Mortality risk factors:
  - ↑ age.
  - Extensive radiographic changes on chest X-ray (CXR).
  - Mechanical ventilation required.
  - Diabetes mellitus.
  - HIV/AIDS.
  - End stage renal disease (ESRD).
- Prevention:
  - BCG vaccination – 80% efficacy, main role is in prevention of severe disease (not routinely given in the UK).

MICRO-facts

The UK guidelines state that TB vaccination should be given to:

- Infants (0–12 months) in areas of the UK with TB incidence of 40/100,000 or greater.
- Infants (0–5 years) with a parent or grandparent born in a country with TB incidence 40/100,000 or greater.
- Child (6–16 years), previously unvaccinated and tuberculin -ve, where parent or grandparent born in a country with TB incidence 40/100,000 or greater.
- Child (0–16 years), tuberculin -ve and previously unvaccinated, born in a country with TB incidence 40/100,000 or greater.
- Child (<16 years), previously unvaccinated and tuberculin -ve, having lived in a country with a TB incidence 40/100,000 or greater, for longer than 3 months.
- Child (<16 years), unvaccinated and tuberculin -ve, who is a contact for a case of respiratory TB.

8.2 EXTRA-PULMONARY TUBERCULOSIS

1. DEFINITION

- TB infection with manifestations in sites other than the lung.
- Extra-pulmonary disease can occur as a direct progression of primary infection or a re-activation of latent TB many years later.

2. EPIDEMIOLOGY AND AETIOLOGY

- Approximately 20% of active TB cases have an extra-pulmonary component and can be classified as extra-pulmonary TB (EPTB).
- The incidence of EPTB is increasing, possibly due to increase in HIV.
- Extra-pulmonary or miliary TB can present with or without pulmonary manifestations and may be the initial presentation (uncommon).

3. PATHOPHYSIOLOGY AND CLINICAL FINDINGS

- Haematogenous spread of bacilli from the pulmonary site of infection.
  - The site of the deposition and granulomas determine the clinical findings.
- Patients with EPTB present with constitutional symptoms, usually alongside respiratory symptoms.

4. TB LYMPHADENITIS

- The lymph nodes are the most common site for EPTB (40% of cases).
  - Cervical > supraclavicular lymph nodes.
  - It is more common in Asian and Black female populations.
- The lymph node enlargement is classically:
  - Painless.
  - Firm.
  - Mobile.
  - Usually without tenderness or discharge.
  - Unilateral or bilateral.
  - Fluctuant.

5. PERICARDIAL TB

- Pericardial infection results from contiguous spread from mediastinal lymph nodes or progression from a latent deposit in the pericardium.
- Pericardial TB can cause:
  - Pericarditis.
  - Pericardial effusion leading to tamponade.
  - Fibrosis leading to cardiac constriction.
- Diagnosis of pericardial TB requires pericardial fluid aspiration or pericardial biopsy.
  - AFB smear and culture.
- Other investigation findings may include:
  - CXR: cardiomegaly.
  - ECG: low voltage with T wave inversion.
  - CT/MRI: pericardial effusion and thickening.

Respiratory Medicine

6. SKELETAL TB

- A type of osteomyelitis, with bacilli deposited in the growth plates of bone where the blood supply is greatest.
- The most common site of skeletal involvement is the vertebral column, especially the lower thoracic and lumbar vertebrae.
  - TB involving the spine is also known as Pott's disease.
- The hip and knee are also common sites of skeletal involvement.
  - TB involving joints is usually mono-articular.
- Clinical features:
  - Dependent on the site of involvement within the skeletal system.
  - Localised pain: insidious onset over weeks to months.
  - Deformity of joint.
  - Cold non-tender swelling (cold abscesses) +/– sinus tract.
  - Pott's disease can cause symptoms secondary to spinal cord compression:
    - Numbness, paraesthesia and weakness below lesion.
    - Incontinence.
    - Paraplegia.
    - Pulmonary features of TB are commonly concurrent with skeletal TB.

7. CNS TB

- The most common presentation of CNS TB is as meningitis, but it can also present as an intercranial tuberculoma or abscess.
  - Sub-meningeal and intra-meningeal deposits of bacilli are called rich foci, which rupture causing meningitis.
- Outcomes of CNS TB are poor, with high level of neurological morbidity and mortality rates at $20-50\%$.
- Clinical features:
  - Fever.
  - Headache.
  - Neck stiffness (meningitis).
  - Behavioural changes.
  - Alterations in consciousness.
  - Focal neurological deficits (often cranial nerve abnormalities).

8. ABDOMINAL TB

- Abdominal TB can involve both the peritoneal cavity and the gastrointestinal tract (TB enteritis), with widespread small granulomatous legions in both.
- TB enteritis is often secondary to ingestion of infected sputum and it causes
  - Caseous necrosis of the intestine, most commonly in the ileocaecal region.

- Mediastinal lymphadenopathy.

Spread to the peritoneum can be via mediastinal lymph node rupture, leading to small tubercles seeded across the peritoneal cavity.

GENITOURINARY TB

Spread forms a primary pulmonary lesion via a haematological route.
Common clinical features are:
- Dysuria
- Haematuria
- Urinary frequency
- Scrotal mass (men)
- Pelvic pain (women).

MILIARY TB

TB is spread from the initial sight in the lung to multiple organ systems, with numerous small lesions of 1–5 mm (see Figure 8.2).
- Haematogenous spread due to erosion of lung lesion into pulmonary vasculature.

The diagnostic efforts for miliary TB focus on the organs most often involved which are shown (in order) in FIgure 8.3:

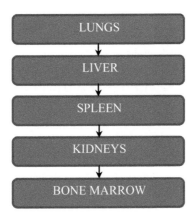

Figure 8.3 Organs most often affected by TB (most often → least often).

Symptoms are usually constitutional:
- Fever
- Anorexia
- Sweats
- Weight loss.

Respiratory Medicine

11. INVESTIGATIONS

- Investigations are the same as for pulmonary TB, with some additional ones dependent on the sight of spread:
    - TB lymphadenitis: consider biopsy or surgical excision of lymph node; send for culture in saline.
    - Skeletal TB: MRI or CT, bone biopsy.
    - CNS TB: Neuroradiology (CT or MRI), CSF examination.
    - Abdominal TB: Peritoneal biopsy and peritoneal fluid analysis.
    - Pericardial TB.
    - Genitourinary TB: KUB ultrasound, urinalysis, urine culture (sterile pyuria: bacilli must be looked for specifically) and consider tissue biopsy.
- The majority of patients with extra-pulmonary TB show characteristic changes of pulmonary TB on CXR.

12. TREATMENT

- The treatment regimens for patients with EPTB are the same as for pulmonary TB (see section 8.3), with a couple of exceptions:
    - Pericardial TB:
        - Glucocorticoid (60 mg prednisolone) – during initiation of treatment with gradual withdrawal after 2–3 weeks.
    - Meningeal TB:
        - Glucocorticoid treatment (as for pericardial TB) with gradual withdrawal over 4–8 weeks.

8.3 TUBERCULOSIS TREATMENT

1. MANAGEMENT OF ACTIVE TB

- Goals of TB treatment are:
    - Achieving cure.
    - Reducing risk of long-term pulmonary damage.
    - Preventing further transmission of TB to others.
- Standard treatment regimens use a minimum of 6 months of antibiotic chemotherapy.
- Four drugs form standard first-line therapy in combination for uncomplicated TB:
    - Rifampicin.
    - Isoniazid.
    - Pyrazinamide.
    - Ethambutol.
    - Pyridoxine (vitamin B6) is usually given alongside antibiotics to reduce the risk of isoniazid-induced peripheral neuropathy.

> ## MICRO-facts
>
> Using the acronym RIPE is an easy way to remember the four mainstay drugs for TB treatment:
>
> - Rifampicin
> - Isoniazid
> - Pyrazinamide
> - Ethambutol.

- Two phases of TB treatment:
  - Intensive phase (2 months): all four of the drugs are given daily.
  - Continuation phase (4 months): only rifampicin and isoniazid are given if patient has responded to the intensive phase and there are no concerns over drug resistance (usual to review drug sensitivities if *M. tuberculosis* cultured).
- Longer continuation phase will be needed for certain patients, such:
  - Meningeal TB: 10 months continuation.
- Patients who are highly infectious (defined as AAFB identified in sputum "smear positive") should remain in isolation, either in a hospital negative pressure room or at home. Patients are considered infectious until they have:
  - Had 3 consecutive AFB negative sputum samples.
  - Been on therapy for at least 2 weeks.
  - Shown clinical improvement.
- Treatment can be unsuccessful and there can be a number of reasons for treatment failure:
  - Poor adherence to medication (most common cause).
  - Poor gastrointestinal absorption.
  - Emergence of drug resistance.
  - Recurrence or relapse.

> ### MICRO-print
> NICE recommends that those who are diagnosed with TB and have recently been on a flight should be reported to the relevant Consultant for Communicable Disease Control (CCDC) and the Health Protection Agency (HPA) if:
>
> - Less than 3 months has elapsed since the flight and the flight was longer than 8 hours and
> - The index case is smear-positive and either:
>   - The index case has multidrug-resistant TB or
>   - The index case coughed frequently during the flight.

2. MANAGEMENT OF LATENT TB

- Patients from a high-risk group with a positive TST/IGRA but no clinical or radiological signs are assumed to have latent TB.
  - An Interferon Gamma Release Assay (IGRA) is more useful in patients with a positive Mantoux or with a previous BCG.
- These patients may require treatment because of the risk of developing active disease within 5 years (overall 15% and up to 50% if HIV positive).
- Consider treatment in adults for:
  - Patients <35 years (older age confers increased hepatotoxicity risk).
  - Any age with HIV.
  - Any age and healthcare worker.
- And:
  - Mantoux positive (>6 mm) without prior BCG.
  - Mantoux positive (>15 mm) or IGRA positive with prior BCG.
- As well as:
  - Patients with evidence of TB scarring on chest X-ray, without a history of adequate treatment.
- There are two regimes recommended by NICE for patients with uncomplicated latent TB infection:
  - Rifampicin + isoniazid daily for 3 months.
  - Isoniazid only daily for 6 months.
  - Pyridoxine is also given in both regimens.

3. MANAGEMENT OF DRUG-RESISTANT TB

- Drug-resistant TB is defined as TB resistant to at least one of the four main drugs.
  - Single agent resistance is treated as follows:

Drug resistance	First 2 months (initial phase)	Continue with (continuation phase)
Isoniazid	Rifampicin, pyrazinamide and ethambutol	Rifampicin and ethambutol for 7 months (up to 10 months for extensive disease)
Pyrazinamide	Rifampicin, isoniazid (with pyridoxine) and ethambutol	Rifampicin and isoniazid (with pyridoxine) for 7 months
Ethambutol	Rifampicin, isoniazid (with pyridoxine) and pyrazinamide	Rifampicin and isoniazid (with pyridoxine) for 4 months
Rifampicin	As for multidrug-resistant TB	As for multidrug-resistant TB

- Multi-drug-resistant TB (MDR-TB) is defined as TB resistant to at least rifampicin and isoniazid (rare in HIV-negative patients).
- Treatment is complex and should always be discussed with a specialist.
- It will generally include a number of second-line drugs (e.g. kanamycin, levofloxacin, linezolid) for periods of up to 24 months.

4. DRUG SIDE EFFECTS

- All first-line drugs can cause general constitutional side effects:
  - Fever
  - Nausea
  - Vomiting
  - Pruritis
  - Anorexia
  - Flushing
  - Diarrhoea
  - Abdominal pains.
- The most common side effects of all the drugs are allergic reactions, including skin rashes.
  - A rare but important skin reaction is the erythema multiforme major rash, Stevens-Johnson syndrome.
    - Almost universally, cases occur in patients who are HIV seropositive.
- Pyrazinamide, rifampicin and isoniazid can cause drug-induced hepatitis, including causing fulminant liver failure.
- Rifampicin:
  - Commonly causes itching in first couple of weeks, so patients should continue medication.
  - Bodily fluids (e.g. urine, tears) become a red/orange colour.
  - Induces cytochrome p450 increasing the clearance of many drugs:
    - ↑ clearance of warfarin, so a dose increase is needed for patients requiring anticoagulation.
  - Increases metabolism of oral contraception so alternative measures need to be taken.
  - Causes a flu-like illness.
- Isoniazid:
  - Peripheral neuropathy + CNS effects.
  - Sideroblastic anaemia.
  - Pyridoxine 10 mg daily usually given as prophylaxis against these side effects.
  - Drug-induced lupus erythematosus.
- Ethambutol:
  - Optic neuritis
  - Red-green colour blindness

- Vertical nystagmus
- Peripheral neuropathy.
- Pyrazinamide:
  - Most common cause of hepatotoxicity.
  - Arthralgia.
  - Interstitial nephritis.

5. COMBINATION DRUG REGIMES

- Using combination fixed dose tablets are advised by the WHO and NICE guidelines for TB treatment.
- The advantages are:
  - Ease of use leading to better treatment adherence.
  - Prevention of drug resistance.
- The combination tablets available in the UK are:
  - Rifater (rifampicin, isoniazid and pyrazinamide).
  - Rifinah (rifampicin and isoniazid).
  - Dosing is based on body weight.

6. MONITORING

- Due to the risk of adverse drug effects and treatment failure patients need monitoring during therapy:
  - LFTs prior to starting therapy; monthly LFTs if baseline is abnormal.
    - Routine monitoring of U&Es and LFTs sometimes needed.
  - Monthly visual checks if taking ethambutol for >2 months.
  - Sputum samples may be undertaken to assess success of treatment regime.
  - CXR after completion of treatment.

8.4 TUBERCULOSIS WORLDWIDE

1. GLOBAL IMPACT AND WHO TARGETS

- 95% of cases and deaths are in developing countries.
  - Asia accounts for 60% of new TB cases globally each year.
  - Proportionally, sub-Saharan Africa has the highest incidence of TB with > 260 per 100,000 per year.
- More than 1/3 of the world's population is infected.
  - Second greatest infectious killer worldwide after HIV/AIDS.
  - In 2013, 9.0 million people fell ill with TB and 1.5 million people died.
- The WHO (World Health Organization) have a number of targets for combating TB, in line with the Millennium Development Goals:
  - 2015: halt and begin to reverse incidence of TB.

- 2015: reduce TB prevalence and deaths by 50% compared to 1990.
- 2050: eliminate TB as a public health problem.
- To achieve these targets the WHO has developed a six-point Stop TB strategy.
    - Pursue high-quality DOTS expansion and enhancement.
    - Address TB-HIV, MDR-TB and the needs of poor and vulnerable populations.
    - Contribute to health system strengthening based on primary health care.
    - Engage all health care providers.
    - Empower people with TB and communities through partnership.
    - Enable and promote research.

2. HIV/AIDS AND TB

- Increases in TB incidence in recent decades have been partly due to the increasing HIV incidence.
    - Impaired system associated with HIV results with increased susceptibility to active TB infections.
    - 15% of those with TB have concurrent HIV.
- Increase in mortality and morbidity in those with HIV co-infection.
    - Individuals infected with HIV and TB are 34 times more likely to develop an active TB infection.
    - TB is the leading killer of HIV infected individuals, causing 25% of HIV/AIDS related deaths.

3. MDR-TB AND XDR-TB

- Worldwide drug resistance is an increasing problem and is a cause of increased morbidity and mortality. It is due to drug regimes that are:
    - Incomplete
    - Incorrect
    - Interrupted.
- MDR-TB is mostly a problem in the developing world, with a relatively small incidence in the developed world (1%), however incidence is increasing in both sectors.
- XDR-TB (extremely drug-resistant TB) is defined as an organism resistant to rifampicin, isoniazid, fluroquinolones and at least one second-line injectable agent (e.g. kanamycin).
    - It is mostly a problem in South-East Asia.
- Isolated total drug resistant strains have been reported in Italy, Iran and India.
- The WHO recommends that all TB drug regimens are DOTS to reduce emerging resistance.

Respiratory Medicine

MICRO-references
WHO Global TB Report 2014:
www.who.int/tb/publications/global_report/gtbr14_main_text.
pdf?ua=1

MICRO-case
A 34-year-old man of Indian origin presents to the GP with a productive cough that has lasted for 3 weeks, along with chest pain. He has a low grade fever and bronchial breathing on auscultation. The GP diagnoses a chest infection and prescribes amoxicillin. The patient fails to respond to amoxicillin after a week. He is subsequently changed to doxycycline and then clarithromycin, with failure to respond to either.

The GP then decides to send off a sputum sample; he notes that the sputum is rusty in colour and blood flecked. On further questioning it emerges that the patient has lost 5 kg since the cough developed, but he does not smoke. He also admits to being a frequent visitor to India on business trips. He has never had a BCG vaccination. The GP sends him for an urgent chest X-ray. The X-ray shows patchy consolidation, hilar lymphadenopathy and a cavitating lesion in the apex of the right lung. A diagnosis of TB is made on radiological and clinical grounds.

The patient is referred to respiratory medicine. The diagnosis is confirmed when acid-fast bacilli are identified in his sputum sample, and 3 weeks later this is further confirmed by culture. He is started on rifampicin, isoniazid, ethambutol and pyrazinamide. He is advised to minimise contact with others during the first 2 weeks of treatment and while symptomatic. The HPA is informed as the patient flew back from India while symptomatic. Three weeks into treatment, the patient produces 3 negative sputum samples and is declared non-infectious. The patient finishes his 6-month treatment course without incident.

Key Points

- A high index of suspicion is needed in patients who may have TB.
- Diagnosis should be considered in those from high-risk groups or returning from abroad.
- TB should be considered in a patient whose respiratory infection does not respond to antibiotic therapy.
- Therapy can be started on clinical and radiological evidence alone, but it is always better to obtain adequate samples for culture first.
- 3 consecutive negative sputum samples are needed before the patient is considered non-infectious if the patient was smear positive prior to treatment.
- TB requires the clinician to complete a notification form to the Health Protection Agency in the UK and DoH.

Respiratory Medicine

9 Bronchiectasis and Cystic Fibrosis

9.1 DEVELOPMENT OF BRONCHIECTASIS

1. DEFINITION

- A disease in which the airways of the lung are thick walled and permanently dilated.
- Bronchial walls are inflamed and irreversibly damaged, which results in frequent infections.

2. EPIDEMIOLOGY

- In the UK the incidence is approximately 1.3 per 100,000.
  - Prevalence increases with age.

3. AETIOLOGY AND RISK FACTORS

- Any insult that causes progressive irreversible bronchial damage can result in bronchiectasis (See Table 9.1).

Table 9.1 **Aetiology of bronchiectasis.**

AETIOLOGY OF BRONCHIAL DAMAGE	CAUSES OF BRONCHIECTASIS
Bronchial obstruction	• Foreign body • Inspissated mucus • Bronchial stenosis • Tumour.

Post infectious	• Prior childhood viral respiratory infection, especially measles.
	• Previous severe pneumonia or mycobacterial infection, for example:
	  • *Bordetella pertussis*.
	  • TB.
	  • *Staphylococcus aureus*.
	  • *Pseudomonas aeruginosa*.

(Continued)

DOI: 10.1201/9781315113937-10

Table 9.1 (*continued*) Aetiology of bronchiectasis.

AETIOLOGY OF BRONCHIAL DAMAGE	CAUSES OF BRONCHIECTASIS
	• *Klebsiella pneumoniae*. • Aspergillus infection. • Swyer-James syndrome. • Post infectious obliterative bronchiolitis. • Unilateral hyper-expanded lung. • Reduced vascularity. • Associated with bronchiectasis.
Immunodeficiency	• HIV/AIDS. • Immunoglobulin deficiency (panhypogammaglobulinaemia or selective deficiencies).
Genetic	• Cystic fibrosis (CF). • Primary ciliary dyskinesia (PCD). • Kartagener's syndrome (subgroup of PCD with situs invertus). • Alpha-1-antitrypsin deficiency (consider if basal emphysema present).
Immunological over-response	• Allergic bronchopulmonary aspergillosis. • Post lung transplant.
Others	• Rheumatoid arthritis. • Yellow nail syndrome. • Idiopathic pulmonary fibrosis. • Inflammatory bowel disease. • Young's syndrome: characterised by azoospermia and sinusitis.

- Cystic fibrosis is the most common cause in the developed world.
- Worldwide HIV/AIDS and infectious causes (especially TB) are more important.
- Some groups have a greater risk of bronchiectasis, including:
  - Women.
  - The elderly.
  - Smokers.

- Those with serious childhood pulmonary infection.
- The immunodeficient.
- Those with inadequately treated pulmonary infection.

MICRO-print

Kartagener's syndrome is a rare autosomal recessive congenital cause of bronchiectasis. It is characterised by the triad:

- Ciliary dyskinesia.
- Dextrocardia.
- Situs inversus (mirroring of major abdominal and thoracic viscera).

It is a cause of recurrent respiratory infections in childhood, which consequently lead to progressive bronchiectasis. The findings on physical examination of the patient are pathognomonic.

PATHOPHYSIOLOGY

- Permanent abnormal widening of the bronchi; this usually occurs due to the repeated cycle shown in Figure 9.1.

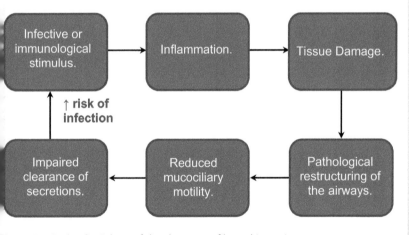

Figure 9.1 Pathophysiology of development of bronchiectasis.

- There is progressive damage due to this process that leads to worsening airflow limitation.
- Pathologically, four different phenotypes of bronchiectasis can be identified:
  - Cylindrical
  - Cystic or saccular
  - Varicose
  - Follicular.

9.2 CLINICAL MANAGEMENT

1. CLINICAL FEATURES

- Clinical features of bronchiectasis are summarised in Table 9.2.

Table 9.2 **Clinical features of bronchiectasis.**

SIGNS	SYMPTOMS	CHEST X-RAY FINDINGS

• Chest:
• Crackles
• Rhonchi
• Scattered wheeze
• Cyanosis
• Clubbing
• Arthritis
• Yellow nails
	• Productive cough:
	  lasting months to years
	• Mucopurulent sputum
	• Dyspnoea
	• Haemoptysis
	• Malaise
	• Recurrent pneumonias
	  (exacerbations)
	• Low-grade fever
	• Pleuritic chest pain
	• Wheeze
	• ↑ Foul-smelling sputum
		• ↑ Pulmonary markings
		  (so-called tramline
		  markings)
		• Atelectasis
		• Honeycomb lung
		• Dilated bronchi
		• Clustered cysts
		• May be normal

2. INVESTIGATIONS

- FBC.
- Serum immunoglobulins: G, A, M and E.
- Serum IgE or skin prick test for *Aspergillus fumigatus*.
- Sputum culture and sensitivity including AAFB culture (to look for *Mycobacterium* spp.).
- Chest X-ray (usually insufficient alone to confirm diagnosis) (see Figure 9.1).
- High-resolution chest CT is the gold standard for diagnosis (see Figure 9.2).
- Sinus X-ray.
- Sweat test (for diagnosis of CF, see section 9.3.6).
- Serum alpha-1-antitrypsin in presence of emphysema.
- Functional antibodies against *Pneumococcus, Haemophilus influenza B* and tetanus.
- Spirometry.

Respiratory Medicine

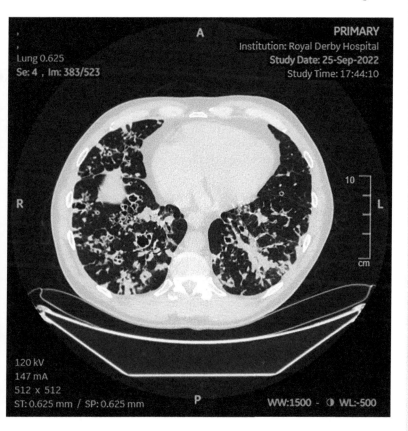

Figure 9.2 Chest CT of a patient with widespread bronchiectasis (CXR and HRCT of bronchiectasis).

DIFFERENTIAL DIAGNOSIS

COPD.
Chronic sinusitis.
Asthma.
Pneumonia.
Chronic bronchitis.
TB.
Gastro-oesophageal reflux disease (GORD).

4. MANAGEMENT

- The management for bronchiectasis differs slightly depending upon the cause.
- Management of non-CF bronchiectasis (see section 9.3.8. for management of CF-bronchiectasis):
  - Antibiotics:
    - Sputum should be sent for bacterial and mycobacterial culture prior to commencing therapy.
    - For acute exacerbations, treatment is with a 10- to 14-day course of one of the following:
      ○ Amoxicillin
      ○ Tetracycline
      ○ A macrolide (e.g. erythromycin)
      ○ Ciprofloxacin (for *Pseudomonas*).
    - Long-term antibiotic therapy should be considered in patients with >3 exacerbations a year. Nebulised colomycin or gentamicin can be used in patients colonised with *Pseudomonas*, and for other patients regime of three times a week oral azithromycin is effective.
  - Chest physiotherapy and pulmonary rehabilitation.
  - Oral mucolytics (e.g. carbocysteine).
  - Nebulised saline (either 0.9% or 7% concentration) as a mucolytic.
  - Short acting β2-agonist bronchodilators (e.g. salbutamol).
  - Inhaled corticosteroids are not routinely used unless there is an associated indication (e.g. asthma/COPD).
  - Prophylactic vaccination against influenza and pneumococcus.
- Lifestyle interventions:
  - Adequate nutrition with supplementation if necessary.
  - Smoking cessation and avoidance of passive smoking.
- Surgery can be considered in some cases:
  - Lung resection in patients with localised disease unresponsive to medical intervention.
  - Bronchial artery embolism if massive haemoptysis occurs.
  - Lung transplantation.

Respiratory Medicine

MICRO-references
The British Thoracic Society (BTS) have produced guidelines for the management of non-CF bronchiectasis:
www.brit-thoracic.org.uk/document-library/guidelines/
bronchiectasis/bts-guideline-for-bronchiectasis-in-adults/

5. COMPLICATIONS

- Repeated infections and progressive deterioration in lung function.
- Empyema.
- Lung abscess.
- Respiratory failure.
- Amyloidosis.

6. PROGNOSIS

- Prognosis varies widely; most patients will have few symptoms and a normal life expectancy.
    - Previous to antibiotic therapy, the majority of patients would die within 5 years.
- Improved survival is associated with:
    - High body mass index (BMI).
    - Up-to-date vaccinations.
- Disease progression is associated with:
    - Colonisation by *P. aeruginosa*.
    - ↑ in number + severity of exacerbations.
    - ↑ CRP.
- Increased mortality is associated with:
    - Hypoxaemia
    - Hypercapnia
    - ↑ dyspnoea
    - Extensive radiological changes.

MICRO-case

A 62-year-old woman visits her GP with a cough productive of mucopurulent sputum. She is a non-smoker with no significant medical problems in her history, and apart from appearing thin, she seems generally well. However the doctor notes that she has been prescribed antibiotics eight times in the last 18 months for bronchitis and has been repeatedly presenting complaining of tiredness. When questioned, the patient admits to having had a persistent productive cough for over a year and getting breathless at times. The GP refers her to a respiratory physician. She does not report a history of heartburn, sinusitis or choking symptoms. She has no evidence of systemic inflammatory disease, no history of TB or whooping cough and has no family history of lung disease. A chest X-ray shows increased lung markings and some dilated airways. An HRCT confirms the presence of dilated bronchi. Blood tests are unremarkable. However when lung function tests are done they show a decreased lung capacity and mild airflow obstruction that improves with the use of bronchodilators. Repeated *continued...*

Respiratory Medicine

continued...
                    sputum cultures grow *Haemophilus influenzae*. A diagnosis of bronchiectasis is made and the patient is started on bronchodilators, carbocysteine, chest physiotherapy and a 3-month course of amoxicillin. Despite an improvement in symptoms, over the next year exacerbations continue. A rotating cycle of month courses of amoxicillin and doxycycline is recommended. This leads to a reduction in sputum volume, purulence and exacerbation frequency.

Key Points

- Although smokers are more likely to develop bronchiectasis, the majority of people who develop it will be non-smokers.
- Diagnosis can be delayed for months or years, with non-specific and mild symptoms often misdiagnosed as bronchitis, asthma or recurrent pneumonia.
- Often a cause for the bronchiectasis cannot be identified.
- Once diagnosed bronchiectasis requires a continuous health maintenance programme, with intermittent aggressive treatment of respiratory infections.

9.3 CYSTIC FIBROSIS

1. DEFINITION

- Cystic fibrosis (CF) is an autosomal recessive multisystem disorder, characterised by frequent respiratory infections and pancreatic insufficiency.

2. EPIDEMIOLOGY

- CF is the most common life limiting genetic condition amongst the Caucasian population.
- 1 / 2500 Caucasian newborns affected.
- Carrier frequency is 1/25.

3. AETIOLOGY AND RISK FACTORS

- CF is caused by a mutation in the Cystic Fibrosis Transmembrane Conductance Receptor (CFTR) gene found on chromosome 7.
- Although there are ~ 1000 different mutations, the most common mutation delta-F508 – accounts for approximately 2/3 of cases of CF.

4. PATHOPHYSIOLOGY

- CFTR is an ATP-responsive chloride channel.
- Other functions include:

Respiratory Medicine

- Regulation of sodium transport across the respiratory epithelium.
- Acting as a cell surface glycoprotein.
- Immune defence.
- Effects of a defective CFTR are described in Figure 9.3:

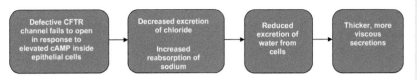

Figure 9.3 Pathophysiological basis of CF.

- **In the airway:**
  - The increased viscosity of the secretions impairs mucociliary clearance.
  - Affected individuals suffer frequent respiratory infections.
  - The cumulative effect of repeated respiratory infections results in progressive lung damage and loss of lung function.
- **In the gastrointestinal (GI) tract:**
  - Increased viscosity of pancreatic secretions leads to reduced secretion from the pancreatic ducts into the small intestine.
    - This causes pancreatic enzyme insufficiency and malabsorption.
  - In the bile ducts, ion transfer is impaired resulting in more concentrated bile which can plug the ducts.
  - Viscous secretions and water movement across the intestinal wall result in intraluminal water deficiency resulting in:
    - Constipation and bowel obstruction.
    - Meconium ileus in the neonate.
- **Infertility**:
  - Infertility in males is caused by the failure of vas deferens development as a direct result of the CFTR mutation.
- **Diabetes**:
  - Cystic fibrosis–related diabetes (CFRD) is caused by progressive pancreatic fibrosis and fatty infiltration, resulting in loss of beta islet cells.

5. CLINICAL FEATURES

- CF may present at any age and the clinical features depend on the age at which it presents.
- **In the neonate:**
  - Detection of increased immunoreactive trypsin in the Guthrie (heel-prick) test.
  - Meconium ileus.
  - Neonatal jaundice.

Respiratory Medicine

- **Infancy and childhood:**
  - Recurrent respiratory infections
  - Failure to thrive
  - Diarrhoea/steatorrhoea
  - Nasal polyps
  - Rectal prolapse
  - Pancreatitis
  - Electrolyte abnormalities
  - Hypoproteinaemia
  - Portal hypertension.
- **Adolescence/adulthood:**
  - Recurrent respiratory infections
  - Bronchiectasis
  - Diabetes
  - Male infertility
  - Portal hypertension
  - Electrolyte abnormality.
- **Signs:**
  - Examination of the older child or adult with CF may reveal:
    - Clubbing.
    - **On auscultation:** crackles and wheeze.
- **Microbial pathogens**
  - ***Pseudomonas aeruginosa:*** This is the most frequently isolated bacteria in adults and is associated with a decrease in lung function.
  - ***Staphylococcus aureus:*** This is the most common pathogen in children with CF.
  - ***Haemophilus influenza:*** Commonly isolated in children but less prevalent in adulthood.
  - ***Burkholderia cepacia:*** A bacterium prevalent amongst CF patients associated with worsening lung function and increased mortality.
  - **Non-tuberculous mycobacteria (NTM):** *M. avium complex, M. abscessus.*
  - ***Stenotrophomonas maltophilia:*** An opportunistic gram-negative bacterium transmitted from contaminated water.

6. INVESTIGATIONS

- **Diagnostic:**
  - **Genetic testing:** Screening for the most common mutations is performed.
  - **Sweat test:** This is the gold standard investigation for CF. A sodium concentration of >60 mmol/L is diagnostic.

- **Monitoring cystic fibrosis:**
  - **Lung function tests:** Spirometry is used in older children, adolescents and adults and demonstrates an obstructive pattern (see Chapter 1: Clinical Assessment).
  - **Blood tests:** FBC, U&E, fasting glucose, LFTs, and vitamin A, D and E levels.
  - **Imaging:** CXR, ultrasound of liver and pancreas.

7. DIFFERENTIAL DIAGNOSIS

- **Respiratory:**
  - Asthma.
  - Allergic bronchopulmonary asthma (ABPA).
  - Primary ciliary dyskinesia/Kartagener's syndrome.
  - Bronchiectasis.
  - Bronchiolitis.
- **Gastro-intestinal:**
  - Coeliac disease.

MICRO-case

You are an SHO working in paediatrics, when Mr and Mrs. Davies bring their 18-month-old son, Alfie, to see you. The child has been lethargic and feeding poorly for the last two days and has a cough. On auscultation, you note widespread crackles and wheeze. This is Alfie's fourth admission to hospital with a respiratory infection. You plot his height and weight on a growth chart and note that he is below the 2nd centile for both. The parents explain their son usually feeds well but remains small. On further history taking, you discover that the parents declined the Newborn Screening (Guthrie) test.

You commence treatment for the acute infection and order a sweat test, which reveals a sodium concentration of 100 mmol/L. Genetic testing demonstrates that the child has the dF508 mutation. The parents are surprised as no one in the family has the condition.

Key Points

- Cystic fibrosis should be suspected in any child demonstrating failure to thrive.
- Pancreatic insufficiency may not be present from birth so growth may be normal at first.
- The Guthrie test is a useful screening tool.
- It is not diagnostic of cystic fibrosis, as it has a high false positive and false negative rate.
- A sweat test should still be performed (sodium concentration >60 mmol/L is diagnostic).

continued...

continued...

- Although the Guthrie test has enabled earlier detection of cystic fibrosis in many cases, you should not exclude the condition from your differential when seeing an older patient.
- Genetic testing is a useful diagnostic tool if the patient has one of the more common CFTR mutations but does not test for all of the possible mutations. Family history may be negative due to the autosomal recessive pattern of inheritance.

8. MANAGEMENT

- The improved survival in cystic fibrosis is partially attributable to the well-structured multidisciplinary approach used in managing the condition.
    - Patients are reviewed regularly and receive input from physicians, specialist nurses, dieticians and physiotherapists, amongst others.

RESPIRATORY MANAGEMENT

- **Airway clearance techniques:**
    - **Physiotherapy:** This is performed for airway clearance usually BD, increasing to QDS if there is an exacerbation (See MICRO-Print, below).
    - **Physical exercise:** This is actively encouraged.
- **Antimicrobial therapy:**
    - **Antibiotic prophylaxis:** Flucloxacillin may be prescribed to prevent *S. aureus* infection.
    - **Antibiotics for infective exacerbations:** See below.
- **Mucolytic agents:**
    - **Nebulised hypertonic saline:** This improves hydration and mobilisation of respiratory secretions.
    - **Nebulised DNase:** This is a recombinant form of human deoxyribonuclease which acts by cleaving neutrophil derived DNA in sputum, reducing viscosity.
    - **Inhaled mannitol:** An osmotic diuretic approved by NICE for use in CF to aid mucociliary clearance.
- **Other inhaled therapies:**
    - **Bronchodilators:** Both short- and long-acting β agonists may be used, delivered via metered dose inhaler or nebuliser.
    - **Inhaled tobramycin:** This anti-pseudomonal drug may reduce the risk of exacerbations.
- **Anti-inflammatory therapy:**
    - **Azithromycin:** This is given for its anti-inflammatory, rather than its anti-microbial, effects.

Respiratory Medicine

- **Prophylaxis:**
  - **Annual influenza vaccination.**
  - **Pneumococcal vaccine.**
- **CFTR modulators:**
  - **Ivacaftor (Kalydeco):** an oral drug that restores functioning of CFTR in patients with the G551D mutation.
    - All patients should undergo genotyping to determine whether they carry the G551D mutation in one of the defective genes.
    - Ivacaftor is not effective in dF508 homozygotes.
  - **Lumacaftor/ivacaftor (Orkambi) and tezacaftor/ivacaftor (Symkevi)** these two combination therapies were approved by NHS England in 2019.
    - Both are suitable for use in dF508 carriers.
  - **Elexacaftor/ivacaftor/tezacaftor (Trikafta):** This triple therapy was approved by NICE as part of a managed access agreement in 2020.
- **Pancreatic insufficiency:**
  - **High-calorie diet:** Patients require around 130% of a normal diet.
  - **Enteric-coated pancreatic enzyme preparations, e.g. Creon:** Match to the lipid content of food so that normal stools are achieved.
  - **Supplements of lipid soluble vitamins:** A, D, E, K.
- **Liver disease:**
  - **Ursodeoxycholic acid:** Improves bile flow.
- **Diabetes:**
  - Prevalence increases with age, with up to 50% of patients over 30 affected.
  - Insulin insufficiency occurs due to decreased β cell mass.
    - A result of fibrosis and atrophy of the pancreas secondary to inflammation and obstruction by viscous secretions.
  - CF-related diabetes is associated with increased mortality.
  - Regular screening for diabetes is performed.
  - Insulin therapy is indicated if diabetes is present.
- **Reproductive:**
  - Most (~97%) men with CF are infertile due to congenital bilateral absence of the vas deferens.
  - Conception is possible via intracytoplasmic sperm injection (ICSI).
  - Reproductive function in women is normal although poor health or nutrition may result in amenorrhoea.
  - Genetic counselling should be offered to couples planning a family.
  - Screening of the partner for carrier status should be considered. If the partner is a carrier, there is a 1 in 2 chance of affected offspring.

Respiratory Medicine

- **Psychological:**
  - Input from clinical psychologists may be required to help patients and their families come to terms with the condition and its implications:
    - Prognosis.
    - High usage of pharmacotherapy and subsequent compliance issues.
    - Fertility.
  - Additional support may be required at diagnosis, in adolescence and towards the end of life.
- **Management of acute exacerbations:**
  - There is some debate about what constitutes an exacerbation in CF. Some indicators may be:
    - Decreased exercise tolerance.
    - Increased cough.
    - Increased sputum.
    - Absence from school or work.
    - Change in appetite/weight loss.
    - Changes on auscultation.
    - Decrease in lung function on spirometry.
  - Exacerbations may be the result of infection with a viral, bacterial or fungal pathogen; or simply the consequence of non-compliance to treatment.
  - **Bacterial infections:** should be managed with antibiotics dictated by the sensitivities of the pathogen.
    - *Pseudomonas aeruginosa*: Oral ciprofloxacin, ± inhaled tobramycin or colistin. IV antibiotics may be indicated.
    - *Burkholderia cepacia*: Oral cotrimoxazole, meropenem or ceftazidime.
  - **IV antibiotics** may be considered in those for whom exacerbations are a frequent occurrence, vascular access may become problematic.
    - An indwelling IV access device may be considered for these patients.
- **Transplant:**
  - A double lung, or heart and lung, transplant may be indicated when there is respiratory failure.
    - It is performed if predicted life expectancy without transplant is <3 years.
  - More than half the CF sufferers on the waiting list will die waiting for a donor.
  - After a lung transplant (for any cause), the five year survival is ~ 50%.

MICRO-print

Physiotherapy in CF

- Active cycle breathing. A cycle of:
    - Breathing control (relaxed breathing).
    - Thoracic expansion exercises (deep breathing).
    - Forced expiration technique (huffs – medium breath in with forced breath out – with breathing control).
    - Repeated until the airway is clear or patient is tired.
- Postural drainage
    - Adjusting body position to encourage drainage of secretions: for example, "tipping" – lying with the head lower than the chest.
- Breathing devices
    - Positive expiratory pressure (PEP) device
    - Oscillating PEP.
- Autogenic drainage
    - A series of breathing exercises aimed at mobilising secretions. 3 phases:
        - A mobilising phase
        - A collecting phase
        - A clearing phase.
    - Breathing at various lung volumes to mobilise secretions at different levels: breathe in, hold breath and breathe out actively ("sighing") until lungs are clear.
- Percussive physiotherapy: for young children
    - A parent/carer performs firm, rhythmical clapping of the child's hest with a cupped hand.

COMPLICATIONS

- **Pulmonary complications:**
    - **Pneumothorax:** spontaneous pneumothorax occurs in 3–4% of CF patients during their lifetime.
    - **ABPA.**
    - **Non-tuberculous mycobacteria.**
    - **Haemoptysis:** commonly occurs, particularly during infective exacerbations
        - Massive haemoptysis: >240 mL within 24 hours or >100 mL daily for several days.
        - Associated with increased age and poor pulmonary function.

Respiratory Medicine

10. PROGNOSIS

- The prognosis for individuals with CF has improved dramatically over the last two decades:
  - The estimated median life expectancy for infants born with the disease is now 40–50 years.
- Lung function decreases with time.
- Colonisation with *Pseudomonas aeruginosa* or *Burkholderia cepacia* can accelerate the destructive processes within the lungs.
- Antibiotic resistance commonly occurs.

MICRO-case

You are a junior doctor working in the CF unit of a busy children's hospital when a 15-year-old schoolgirl comes in for her three-month review with her parents. Her mother is concerned because Lucy has been coughing more often than she used to and struggles to play a full 70-minute game of hockey, her favourite sport.

Spirometry reveals that her FEV$_1$ and FVC have both deteriorated since her last review 3 months before.

You take sputum samples and commence antibiotic therapy, according to the local guidelines.

When the results of the sputum are returned, you are surprised to find that they are negative for any causative organisms.

When Lucy returns to clinic, you ask to see her alone and she confesses that she has stopped using her nebuliser and performing her physiotherapy exercises. She explains that she hates feeling different to the other girls in her school and wants to exert some control of her own life.

You decide to refer her to a psychologist to discuss the issues surrounding her non-compliance.

Key Points

- Spirometry is a useful tool for monitoring changes in lung function.
- Symptomatic changes or changes in function should be investigated fully.
- Empirical antibiotic therapy should be commenced in patients with exacerbations of CF:
  - Liaison with microbiology is necessary to select appropriate antibiotic therapy.
- Poor compliance is an enduring problem in CF, particularly during the adolescent years:
  - Psychology input can be very beneficial.
- An MDT approach underlies success in managing cystic fibrosis

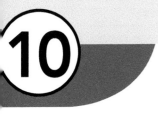

Sarcoidosis

DEFINITION

- Sarcoidosis is a systemic inflammatory condition characterised by the presence of non-caseating granulomas in affected organs.
- Sarcoidosis most commonly affects the lung and intrathoracic lymph nodes, but can affect any system including the liver, heart, skin and eyes.

EPIDEMIOLOGY

- In the UK incidence of sarcoidosis is around 1 in $10,000$.
- It most commonly presents between the ages of 20 *to* 50 years.
- 50% of cases have pulmonary involvement only.
- The disease is more common in Afro-Caribbean and female patients.

PATHOPHYSIOLOGY

- The cause of sarcoidosis is unknown.
- It has been postulated that there may be genetic or infective triggers (particularly *Mycobacterium* spp. since there are similar pathological findings).
- Biopsy of lesions shows granulomatous tissue (organised collections of epithelioid cells) with no necrosis or infective pathogens.

CLINICAL FEATURES

- Patients have no symptoms in 5% of cases.
- Clinical features are listed in Table 10.1.

Table 10.1 **Clinical features of sarcoidosis.**

Pulmonary	• Cough • Shortness of breath on exertion • Chest pain
Systemic	• Fever and sweats • Weight loss • Fatigue

(Continued)

DOI: 10.1201/9781315113937-11

Table 10.1 (*continued*) Clinical features of sarcoidosis.

Skin	• Erythema nodosum • Lupus pernio • Skin nodules
Eyes	• Uveitis • Conjunctivitis
Cardiac	• Complete heart block • Ventricular arrhythmia • Congestive cardiac failure
Neurological	• Cranial nerve palsy (commonly CN VII) • Peripheral neuropathies • Seizures

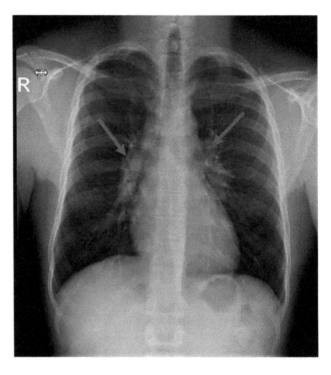

Figure 10.1 A chest X-ray showing classical bilateral hilar lymphadenopathy and infiltrate of a patient with sarcoidosis.

MICRO-print
Löfgren Syndrome
A triad of bilateral hilar lymphadenopathy, erythema nodosum and arthritis. It usually presents with subacute symptoms but carries an excellent prognosis and will normally not require treatment.

5. INVESTIGATIONS

- **Chest X-ray (CXR):**
  - Changes on CXR can be classified into stages (see Table 10.2), however they can correlate poorly to symptom burden.

Table 10.2 **Stages of sarcoidosis.**

Stage I	Hilar or mediastinal nodal enlargement only (bilateral hilar lymphadenopathy or BHL)
Stage II	Nodal enlargement and parenchymal disease (See Figure 10.1)
Stage III	Parenchymal disease only
Stage IV	Pulmonary fibrosis (See Figure 10.2)

- **CT chest**
  - More sensitive than CXR for detecting parenchymal changes.
  - Able to accurately delineate mediastinal and hilar lymphadenopathy.
  - May demonstrate pleural and subpleural and fissural nodules.
  - Fibrotic changes in stage IV disease.
- **Pulmonary function tests (PFTs):**
  - Abnormal lung function is found in 20% of stage I disease, but highly variable with stage 2–4 disease.
  - Both obstructive and restrictive features can be found:
    - Restrictive defects occur a result of pulmonary fibrosis.
    - Obstructive defects may be the result of a number of processes:
      - ○ Due to narrowing of bronchial walls.
      - ○ Peribronchiolar fibrosis.
      - ○ Small airways disease.
      - ○ Compression by enlarged lymph nodes.
  - FEV_1, FVC and T_{LCO} are used to monitor disease progression.

Respiratory Medicine

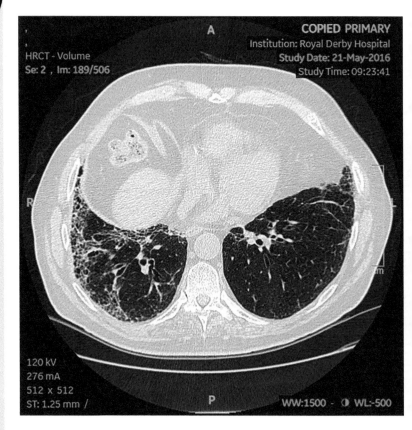

Figure 10.2 A CT chest showing honeycomb changes in periphery and bases of lung characteristic of stage IV sarcoidosis.

- **Biopsy:**
    - The main differential diagnoses are lung cancer, lymphoma and tuberculosis.
    - Biopsy is often not required in cases where there is strong clinical evidence to support the diagnosis in stage I or stage II disease (e.g. Lofgren's syndrome).
    - Endobronchial ultrasound guided aspiration of mediastinal or hilar lymphadenopathy is the preferred technique as it is relatively safe and provides a high diagnostic yield.
    - Transbronchial biopsy (bronchoscopically guided sampling of abnormal lung parenchyma) can be used if there is no lymphadenopathy but carries significant risk of pneumothorax and haemorrhage.
    - Endobronchial biopsies (sensitivity only 40%).

- Some mediastinal nodes cannot be accessed with EBUS and mediastinoscopy or VATS can be undertaken to sample these if diagnostic uncertainty (e.g. sarcoid vs. lymphoma).
- Peripheral lymph nodes or skin lesions/liver/renal tissue can be sampled if thought to be involved.
- **Angiotensin converting enzyme (ACE) levels:**
  - Sensitivity 60% and specificity 70%.
  - A normal level does not rule out sarcoidosis, nor does a raised level confirm the diagnosis.
  - May improve with response to treatment.
- **Serum calcium and 24-hour urinary calcium:**
  - Hypercalcaemia is seen in 5–10% of patients, and hypercalciuria is present in 40–62%.
  - Hypercalcaemia and hypercalciuria can cause renal calculi, and nephrocalcinosis leading to renal failure.
- **ECG:**
  - Refer for cardiology assessment if there is any indication of conduction abnormalities, or a history of syncope.
  - Cardiac MRI or PET scanning may be required.
- **Eye examination:**
  - Ophthalmic involvement is seen in 10 – 50% of patients with sarcoidosis.
- **Liver function tests (LFTs):**
  - Up to 35% of patients with sarcoidosis will have abnormal LFTs.

6. DIFFERENTIAL DIAGNOSIS

- Tuberculosis
- Lymphoma
- Lung cancer
- Atypical infection
- Aspergillosis
- Pneumoconiosis
- Granulomatosis with polyangiitis.

7. MANAGEMENT

- **Stage I:**
  - Treatment of stage I disease is not indicated if asymptomatic.
  - Arthralgia can be treated with simple analgesia such as NSAIDs.
  - Oral steroids can be given if systemic symptoms are severe (e.g. sweats, fatigue).
- **Stages II and III:**
  - Asymptomatic patients with stable, mildly abnormal lung function do not need treatment.

- Symptomatic or progressive disease is treated with oral corticosteroid (such as prednisolone) for 6 to 24 months.
- Patients that do not respond to steroids can be considered for immuno-suppressive treatment such as methotrexate.

- **Stage IV:**
  - Patients with stage IV disease often respond poorly to steroid and immunosuppressive therapy.
- **Follow-up:**
  - Follow up in clinic every 3 to 6 months for the first 2 years to monitor PFTs, symptom burden and response to treatment.
  - Patients with persistent disease should be seen in clinic indefinitely.

MICRO-facts

Steroid Therapy Considerations

- With long-term prednisolone use, advise patients about symptoms of hyperglycaemia and weight gain.
- Counsel patients about the risk of adrenal suppression.
- Osteoporosis is a complication of long-term steroid treatment, and bone mineral density monitoring and bisphosphonate (or other) therapy should be considered.

---

8. COMPLICATIONS

- **Treatment related:**
  - Steroid-related complications (see MICRO-Facts, above).
  - Immunosuppressant therapy causing opportunistic infection.
- **Pulmonary:**
  - Pulmonary arterial hypertension.
  - Fibrosis.
- **Extra-pulmonary:**
  - Fatal arrhythmias, heart block and congestive heart failure.
  - Renal failure and renal calculi.
  - Peripheral neuropathy, cranial nerve palsy and intracranial lesions.
  - Glaucoma, cataracts, optic atrophy and vision loss.
- **Systemic:**
  - Fatigue
  - Depression.

9. PROGNOSIS

There are high rates of spontaneous remission (See Table 10.3).
- $10 - 20\%$ of patients have permanent end organ damage.
- Overall mortality of $1 - 5\%$.

Respiratory Medicine

Table 10.3 **Rates of spontaneous remission in sarcoidosis.**

	Spontaneous Remission Rates
Stage I	50–90%
Stage II	40–70%
Stage III	10–20%
Stage IV	0%

MICRO-case
You are a respiratory consultant working in the outpatient department. A 40-year-old woman has been referred urgently due to a mass seen on her chest X-ray. She had seen her GP 6 months ago for shortness of breath on climbing stairs and persistent cough. She had been initially diagnosed with asthma and treated with inhalers but had become increasingly short of breath and tired, to the extent she can no longer work as a teacher.

On further questioning, she has also had painful swollen joints in her hands, painful nodular rash on her legs, and has been taking drops for dry eyes. The CXR requested by her GP demonstrates bilateral hilar lymphadenopathy (BHL) and pulmonary infiltrates. You request further investigations. CT chest confirmed bilateral hilar and mediastinal lymphadenopathy, as well as small nodules throughout the parenchyma. PFTs reveal a reduced FEV_1 at 78% predicted, with a normal T_{LCO}. Histology from trans-bronchial biopsy shows a non-caseating granuloma. You diagnose her with stage II sarcoidosis. As she is symptomatic, you start her on 40 mg of prednisolone a day for 4 weeks, and then to be gradually reduced to a maintenance dose. You organise an ECG and refer to an ophthalmologist for assessment.

You see her in clinic in 3 months' time for review. Her shortness of breath, rash and joint pain are much better, and her FEV_1 is now normal. You decide to keep her on the maintenance dose of prednisolone and see her again in 3 months' time for repeat PFTs and clinical review.

Key Points
- Sarcoidosis is most common between the ages of 20 and 50, and is more common in females than males.
- Sarcoidosis can affect any system of the body, and a detailed history should be taken to elucidate any extra-pulmonary symptoms.
- Decision to treat is based on symptoms, radiological findings and PFTs.

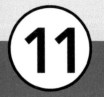

11 Interstitial Lung Disease and Vasculitis

11.1 CLASSIFICATION OF INTERSTITIAL LUNG DISEASES

- The term interstitial lung disease (ILD) encompasses a large group of at least 200 disorders affecting the pulmonary parenchyma, the majority of which are rare.
- "Interstitial lung disease" and "pulmonary fibrosis" are not interchangeable terms, and where appropriate it is best to use the most precise terms/diagnosis.
- However, precise diagnosis can be very difficult and some types of ILD may be termed "unclassifiable".
- ILD is classified according to the flowchart in Figure 11.1.

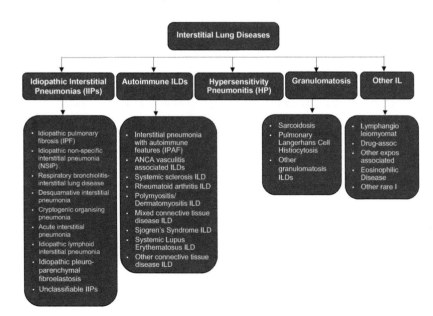

Figure 11.1 Classification of ILD.

DOI: 10.1201/9781315113937-12

11.2 IDIOPATHIC PULMONARY FIBROSIS (IPF)

1. DEFINITION

- Chronic, progressive fibrosing interstitial pneumonia of unknown aetiology limited to the lungs and associated with histopathological or radiological features of usual interstitial pneumonitis (UIP).
- UIP is a pathological entity defined by a combination of:
    1. Patchy interstitial fibrosis.
    2. Fibroblastic foci on histological samples.
    3. Architectural change – chronic scarring and honeycomb lung.
- There are a number of CT scan findings that correlate strongly with UIP pathology, and so a CT scan may report UIP even though it is strictly a pathological finding.
- The term UIP is often used interchangeably with IPF. However, other conditions can result in the same pathological changes e.g. drug toxicity, connective tissue disease, asbestosis.
- Historically, the condition was termed "cryptogenic fibrosing alveolitis", but this term was deprecated with the realisation that it is a fibrotic rather than an inflammatory disease.

2. EPIDEMIOLOGY

- In the UK the incidence is 7 per 100,000 patient years. There are over 5000 cases diagnosed each year.
- The rate of IPF is higher in men.
- The disease most commonly presents in the sixth and seventh decade.
- It is unusual for patients under age 50 years to have IPF in the absence of underlying connective tissue disease (e.g. systemic sclerosis).
- Most patients will have a smoking history.

3. AETIOLOGY

- The cause of IPF is unknown but potential triggers of injury could include:
    - Environmental dust
    - Smoking
    - Viral infection
    - Chronic aspiration.
- Family history may suggest familial pulmonary fibrosis. However, this is rare and associated with < 5% of patients with IPF.
- The pathophysiological process underlying IPF is described in Figure 11.2.

Respiratory Medicine

4. PATHOPHYSIOLOGY

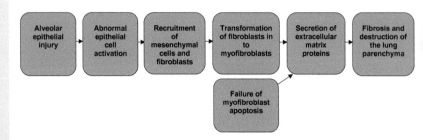

Figure 11.2 Pathophysiology of IPF.

5. CLINICAL FEATURES

- **Symptoms:**
  - Typically present for 6 to 9 months before presentation.
  - Insidious onset:
    - Increasing breathlessness
    - Dry cough.
  - Constitutional symptoms:
    - Malaise
    - Weight loss
    - Fatigue.
- **History:**
  - Occupational history: Exposure to dusts such as metal, asbestos and wood.
  - Symptoms of reflux: Gastroesophageal reflux disease is thought to be associated with IPF.
  - Drugs that cause fibrosis include amiodarone, nitrofurantoin and methotrexate.
  - Family history: Familial pulmonary fibrosis (associated with less than 5% of patients with IPF).
  - Features of connective tissue disease suggest this is not idiopathic.
- **Signs:**
  - Fine basal end-inspiratory crackles on auscultation.
  - Finger clubbing: in 25 – 50% of patients.
  - Signs of cor pulmonale may be present in advanced disease.

MICRO-facts

Cor Pulmonale

- Right heart failure caused by pulmonary hypertension.
- Clinical features:
  - Pedal oedema
  - Raised JVP
  - Hepatomegaly
  - Ascites.
- Congestive heart failure may occur with co-existent left ventricular symptoms:
  - Shortness of breath
  - Bibasal crackles on auscultation
  - Cardiac wheeze
  - Orthopnoea
  - Paroxysmal nocturnal dyspnoea.

INVESTIGATIONS

- **Blood tests** may reveal an specific diagnosis other than IPF (applicable for investigation in all patients with fibrosis):
  - Rheumatoid factor/anti-CCP antibodies.
  - ESR/CRP.
  - ANCA.
  - ANA (if positive, check anti-ENA and anti-dsDNA antibodies).
  - Anti-Scl70 and anti-Jo-1 antibodies.
  - Aspergillus and avian precipitins.
- **CXR:**
  - Changes are not specific for IPF and may be normal in early disease.
  - Peripheral or basal reticular shadowing: a complex network of curvilinear opacities that diffusely involve the lung (See Figure 11.3).
- **High-resolution CT (HRCT):**
  - Findings are more specific than CXR for diagnosis.
  - Sensitivity is high for UIP, replacing the need for lung biopsy in most patients.
  - Predominately subpleural and basal reticular change.
  - Honeycombing (characteristic feature) with or without traction bronchiectasis.

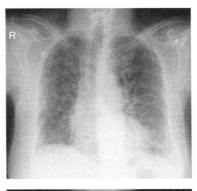

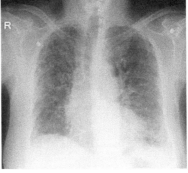

Figure 11.3 Chest X-ray of patient with pulmonary fibrosis. This shows classical signs bilateral, peripheral, and basal reticulonodular infiltrate – as well as reduced lung volume

- **Pulmonary function tests:**
  - Usually restrictive spirometry:
    - Reduced FEV_1 and FVC with normal or high FEV_1/FVC ratio.
  - Reduced vital capacity and transfer factor.
  - Hypoxia on exertion.
    - Occurs at rest in later disease.
- **Biopsy:**
  - Biopsy may be needed if there is diagnostic doubt.
  - Obtained via thoracoscopy or video assisted thoracoscopic surgery (VATS) procedure.
  - Transbronchial biopsy provides poor diagnostic yield due to the small size of sample. A newer technique of cryobiopsy that can provide larger samples is not yet widely used.
  - Histological appearance is of:
    - Areas of scarring and fibrosis alternating with areas of normal parenchyma.
    - Fibroblast foci consisting of sub-epithelial areas of proliferating fibroblasts and myofibroblasts.
    - Cystic fibrotic airspaces make up the "honeycomb" changes.

- A diagnosis of IPF is only made after multidisciplinary correlation of clinical, radiology +/- pathology findings, and is termed definite, probable or possible depending on the exact combination of findings.

MANAGEMENT

- **Clinical assessment:**
  - Clinical review can be tailored to the symptoms/severity of the condition.
  - Patients should have their Tlco and (F)VC measured each visit.
  - Decline in lung function defined as a sustained fall in VC/Tlco of 10−15% should prompt consideration of pharmacological treatment.
  - Patients who are highly symptomatic at presentation should also be considered for pharmacological treatment.
- **Pharmacological therapy:**
  - **Pirfenidone:**
    - Oral immunosuppressant that likely suppresses fibroblast activity.
    - Licensed in the UK for individuals with an FVC 50−80% of predicted.
    - Consider stopping if FVC continues to fall >10% in 12 months.
    - Can slow FVC decline, improve progression free survival and improve exercise tolerance.
    - May lead to improvement in all-cause mortality.
  - **Nintedanib:**
    - Oral tyrosine kinase inhibitor which reduces fibrogenic growth factors.
    - Licensed similar to pirfenidone but recently approved for use with $FVC > 80\%$.
    - Reduces disease progression, time to first exacerbation, and may improve survival.
  - **Corticosteroids:**
    - Although used extensively in the past, evidence suggests they are not effective since IPF is not an inflammatory condition. May be used as a short course in patients with an acute exacerbation of symptoms.
- **Supportive therapy:**
  - **Long-term oxygen therapy:**
    - Patients with severe hypoxia should be treated with supplementary oxygen.
    - There is no proven long-term survival benefit.
    - May reduce risk of cor pulmonale and pulmonary hypertension.
    - Improves exercise tolerance.
  - **Pulmonary rehabilitation:**
    - Pulmonary rehabilitation provides a combination of breathing exercises, exercise training, patient education, psychiatric and social support.
    - It can improve quality of life and exercise tolerance.

Respiratory Medicine

- **Transplant**
    - Patients should be considered for transplant if they are:
        - Under the age of 65.
        - Have failed trial of treatment.
    - With one of:
        - *TLCO* < 40%.
        - Progressive FVC decline > 10% within 6 months.
        - Resting hypoxia.
        - Pulmonary hypertension.

8. PROGNOSIS

- Median survival is 3–5 years.
- Patients who receive single lung transplant:
    - 1 year actuarial survival of 80%.
    - 3 year survival of 55%.
- **Factors associated with poor prognosis:**
    - 10% decline of FVC over 6 months:
        - 2.4-fold increased risk of death.
    - Pulmonary hypertension:
        - Increased symptoms.
        - Increased 1-year mortality.
        - More likely to have complications from lung transplant.
    - Oxygen desaturation below 88% on a 6-minute walk test:
        - 4-year survival of 35% compared to a survival of 69% in those who did not desaturate below 88%.
    - Male sex.
    - Older age.
    - Multiple hospital admissions.
    - Low TLCO.

11.3 OTHER IDIOPATHIC INTERSTITIAL PNEUMONIAS

1. NONSPECIFIC INTERSTITIAL PNEUMONIA (NSIP)

- NSIP is an idiopathic interstitial pneumonia that is not pathologically compatible with usual, desquamative or acute interstitial pneumonia (see below).
- Patients with NSIP have a greater response to steroids and a better prognosis than those with IPF.
- NSIP presents in a younger population, typically those in the fifth and sixth decades.
- Often associated with connective tissue disease.
- Presentation:

- Similar manner to IPF:
  - Cough
  - Dyspnoea of gradual onset.
- Examination findings:
  - Inspiratory crackles
  - Sometimes finger clubbing.
- HRCT findings differ from IPF and show diffuse ground glass change (See Figure 11.4).
- Histology is variable, and can be characterised as either:
  - Cellular: interstitial inflammation with no fibrosis, associated with good prognosis.
  - Fibrotic: interstitial fibrosis more homogenous than in UIP and with no characteristic fibroblastic foci.
- Treatment is predominately with steroids, and sometimes other immunosuppressants.

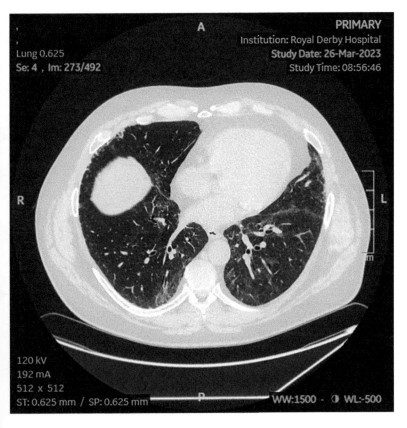

Figure 11.4 High-resolution chest CT of patient with NSIP showing diffuse ground glass changes.

2. CRYPTOGENIC ORGANISING PNEUMONIA (COP)

- In COP alveolar buds fill with granulation tissue, which is made up of a mix of myofibroblasts and connective tissue.
- Patients present with a short history (<3 months) of cough and dyspnoea, often accompanied by systemic features such as weight loss, malaise and fever.
- HRCT shows either areas of consolidation with ground glass change or a solitary nodule.
- COP is treated with a tapered course of prednisolone over several months.
  - Patients usually respond promptly to steroids.
  - May relapse as the dose is reduced.
  - 6 to 12 months of treatment is normally required.

3. RESPIRATORY BRONCHIOLITIS–ASSOCIATED INTERSTITIAL LUNG DISEASE (RB-ILD)

- Proliferation of bronchiolar pigmented macrophages in the terminal bronchioles causing interstitial lung disease.
- RB-ILD occurs in smokers (>30-year pack history).
- More common in males.
- Presents in the fourth to fifth decades.
- Patients present with mild dyspnoea and cough.
- HRCT demonstrates ground glass changes with thick-walled airways and centrilobular nodules.
- Smoking cessation is essential to treatment.
- Steroids may provide some benefit.

4. LYMPHOID INTERSTITIAL PNEUMONIA (LIP)

- Interstitial pneumonia caused by lymphoid infiltrates.
- Patients present with gradual onset of dyspnoea over several years.
  - May also have a history of fever or weight loss.
- LIP is associated with:
  - Connective tissue disease (e.g. Sjögren's syndrome).
  - Autoimmune disease (e.g. myasthenia gravis, pernicious anaemia).
  - Immunodeficiency (e.g. common variable immunodeficiency, HIV).
- HRCT shows ground glass change and can demonstrate nodules or lung cysts.
- Steroids are the mainstay of treatment.
- One-third of patients progress to chronic fibrosis.

5. DESQUAMATIVE INTERSTITIAL PNEUMONIA (DIP)

- Caused by abnormal proliferation of pigmented macrophages as in RB-ILD, however in DIP they are found throughout the alveolar air spaces.

Respiratory Medicine

- Highly associated with smoking.
- Treatment is the same as RB-ILD.
- Prognosis is good.

6. ACUTE INTERSTITIAL PNEUMONIA

- Diffuse alveolar damage and fibrosis associated with rapid onset of dyspnoea followed by respiratory failure.
- CXR shows bilateral diffuse airway shadowing, which can spare heart borders and hilum.
- HRCT shows ground glass change progressing to reticulation and cystic change.
- Lung biopsy demonstrates diffuse alveolar damage comprising of hyaline membranes, necrosis of alveolar lining cells, fibroblastic tissue, scarring and honeycombing – but is rarely done as patients are usually too ill.
- Treatment is supportive, and level 2/3 care may be offered in patients with single organ failure, although prognosis is extremely poor with 70% mortality at 3 months.
- High-dose steroids (e.g. IV methylprednisolone) and antibiotics are often used.
- It is important to look carefully for evidence of underlying connective tissue disease or opportunistic infection (e.g. PJP), which might require specific treatments.

11.4 HYPERSENSITIVITY PNEUMONITIS (HSP)

1. DEFINITION

- Previously called extrinsic allergic alveolitis.
- Immunological reaction within the lung in response to inhaled antigens (see Table 11.1) that can have variable clinical presentation.

2. EPIDEMIOLOGY

- Variable depending on antigen and time of year.
    - Farmer's lung 12–2300 per 100,000.
    - Bird fancier's lung 20–20,000 per 100,000.

3. AETIOLOGY

- Due to exposure to organic and inorganic airborne antigens.
- Certain occupations carry a higher risk – agriculture and cattle workers, bird and poultry handlers, veterinary work and animal handling, grain and flour processing, construction.

Respiratory Medicine

Table 11.1 **Causes of EAA.**

Form of EAA	Precipitant/Antigen
Farmers' lung	Mouldy hay (*Saccharopolyspora rectivirgula*)
Bird fancier's lung	Avian proteins
Cheese worker's lung	Cheese mould (*Penicillium casei*)
Malt worker's lung	Mouldy malt (*Aspergillus clavatus*)
Mushroom worker's lung	Mushroom compost (actinomycetes)
Hot tub lung	*Mycobacterium avium*
Chemical worker's lung	Many antigens during manufacture of plastics, rubber etc.

4. PATHOPHYSIOLOGY

- Types III and IV hypersensitivity reactions identified (see MICRO-Print, below).
- Possibly TH1 pathway is dominant upon interaction with inhaled antigen.
- IgG precipitins may be detected.

MICRO-print

Hypersensitivity Reactions

Undesirable reactions produced by the host immune system to antigens. Type III and IV are implicated in EAA.

- **Type I – Allergy:** Fast, IgE mediated response. Occurs in minutes. E.g. asthma, anaphylaxis.
- **Type II – Cytotoxic:** IgM/IgG binds to a target (host) cell, triggering destruction of that cell. E.g. autoimmune haemolytic anaemia, Goodpasture's syndrome.
- **Type III – Immune complex:** IgG binds to a soluble antigen, forming immune complexes which are deposited on tissues and initiate inflammation e.g. post streptococcal glomerulonephritis.
- **Type IV – Delayed-type hypersensitivity:** T helper cells (Th1 cells) are activated by antigen presenting cells. Later exposure to that antigen activates macrophages and an inflammatory response. E.g. contact dermatitis, Mantoux test.

---

5. CLINICAL FEATURES

- Acute form:
    - Symptom onset within 4 hours of exposure.
    - Can resolve within hours to weeks if antigen exposure is ceased.
- Disease can be insidious, leading to progressive symptoms.
- **Symptoms:**
    - Cough
    - Breathlessness
    - Fever
    - Malaise
    - Weight loss.
- **Signs:**
    - Crackles audible on auscultation.
    - Clubbing can be present in progressive disease.
    - Respiratory failure in late disease.

6. INVESTIGATIONS

- **Serum precipitins**
    - Precipitins against relevant antigen can be raised, e.g. avian, but commercially available assay may not be available for many antigens.
- **CXR**
    - Can be normal especially in acute EAA if timing is incorrect in relation to antigen exposure.
    - In chronic disease, nodular-reticular change visible in mid and upper zones.
- **HRCT**
    - Combination of centrilobular lung nodules, ground glass changes, air trapping and fibrosis in late stages (mainly mid-zone).
- **Pulmonary function tests**
    - Reduced Tlco in chronic disease.
    - Spirometry is either restrictive or mixed obstructive – restrictive pattern.
- **Inhalation challenge testing**
    - Exposure to offending environment with antigen with clinical assessment including real-time lung function and radiology assessment.
    - Provided by specialist centres.
- **BAL**
    - Lymphocytosis evident.
    - CD4+/CD8+ ratio < 1.
    - BAL neutrophilia and eosinophilia also can be present.

- **Biopsy**
  - Surgical lung biopsy required in diagnostic doubt.
  - Small non-caseating ill-defined granulomas seen along bronchioles.
  - Bronchocentric distribution of mononuclear cell infiltration.
  - Peribronchiolar fibrosis with Schaumann bodies.
- Diagnosis is usually made in a multidisciplinary setting based on integration of clinical, serological, radiological and pathological features.

7. MANAGEMENT

- Removal from antigen.
- Change in work practice if relevant.
- Respiratory protective masks may help.
- Corticosteroid therapy (may not reverse process in progressive HSP with end stage fibrosis) with prednisolone at 0.5 mg/kg with tapering over 4–6 months.

8. PROGNOSIS

- Cessation of antigen exposure +/– corticosteroid therapy in most patients will lead to good resolution of EAA changes.
- In severe disease resolution may take years.
- Disease may sometimes progress despite elimination of culprit antigen, but should prompt reconsideration of diagnosis.

11.5 ILD ASSOCIATED WITH NON-PULMONARY CONDITIONS

1. DRUGS

- Interstitial lung disease can occur as a result of drug side effects:
  - Amiodarone
  - Bleomycin
  - Methotrexate
  - Nitrofurantoin.

2. SYSTEMIC RHEUMATIC CONDITIONS

- Rheumatoid arthritis
- SLE
- Systemic sclerosis
- Ankylosing spondylitis
- Dermatomyositis
- Polymyositis.

Respiratory Medicine

3. VASCULITIS: SEE SECTION 11.6

MICRO-case

You are working as a respiratory physician when a 70-year-old gentleman comes to see you after a GP referral. He has suffered with shortness of breath which he first noticed around 6 months ago. Over the last 6 months, it has worsened progressively, limiting his exercise tolerance significantly. He has also lost around a stone in weight over the same time period. He does not have a cough or wheeze. On examination, you note fine bibasal inspiratory crackles on auscultation.

Chest X-ray showed basal reticular shadowing. An HRCT demonstrated honeycombing. Spirometry reveals an FEV_1/FVC ratio of 0.9 but both values are reduced. Tlco is also reduced. All blood tests are normal.

His medication history is reviewed: he takes amlodipine for blood pressure and simvastatin for high cholesterol but no other medications. He formerly worked as a maths teacher and has never been exposed to asbestos or other dusts.

Having excluded all other causes for pulmonary fibrosis, you diagnose probable IPF, which is later confirmed at a multidisciplinary meeting. Due to the characteristic HRCT changes, biopsy is not indicated. Treatment with nintedanib is recommended.

Key Points

- Pulmonary fibrosis may have an insidious onset.
- Progressive shortness of breath is the most common presenting feature.
- Honeycombing on HRCT is characteristic of UIP.
- Biopsy may be required in cases where the diagnosis is not evident from HRCT alone.
- Good history taking is essential to establish the cause of fibrosis, e.g. occupational (see Chapter 16 for more information), drug induced, systemic and familial disease.

11.6 VASCULITIS AND THE LUNG

- The systemic vasculitides are a heterogeneous group of disorders characterised by an inflammatory destructive process affecting blood vessels.
- The lung is frequently involved with various clinical presentations.
- These vasculitides may be primary or associated with other systemic disease such as connective-tissue disease.
- The primary vasculitides affecting the lung are often associated with ANCA (antinuclear cytoplasmic antibody) positivity.

- Indirect immunofluorescent staining patterns differentiate two main types:
  - Cytoplasmic ANCA (c-ANCA) are primarily, but not exclusively, directed against proteinase 3 (PR-3).
  - Perinuclear ANCA (p-ANCA) are most commonly directed against myeloperoxidase (MPO).
- The ANCA blood test is very important in diagnosis, classification and monitoring response to treatment.

11.7 EOSINOPHILIC GRANULOMATOSIS WITH POLYANGIITIS (EGPA)

1. DEFINITION AND EPIDEMIOLOGY

- An eosinophil-rich and granulomatous necrotising vasculitis affecting small to medium-sized vessels in the upper and lower respiratory tract.
- Previously termed Churg-Strauss syndrome.
- Carries an association with asthma and should therefore be considered in the presence of a blood eosinophilia.
- It is the rarest of all the anti-neutrophil cytoplasmic auto-antibody (ANCA) vasculitides with an epidemiology of 1–3 cases per million, with a slight male predominance.

2. AETIOLOGY AND PATHOPHYSIOLOGY

- Aetiology and pathogenesis is unknown.
- An association with inhaled glucocorticoid therapy, leukotriene modifying agents and omalizumab has been noted but may reflect unmasking of EGPA with reduction of oral corticosteroid therapy.
- There are 3 pathological phases to the disease that classically occur sequentially (See Figure 11.5).

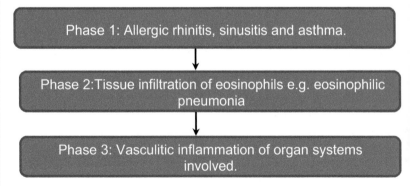

Figure 11.5 Pathophysiology of EPGA.

Phase 1: Allergic rhinitis, sinusitis and asthma.

Phase 2: Tissue infiltration of eosinophils e.g. eosinophilic pneumonia

Phase 3: Vasculitic inflammation of organ systems involved.

Respiratory Medicine

3. CLASSIFICATION

- The presence of 4 or more of the following criteria as defined by the American College of Rheumatology:
    - Asthma.
    - Peak peripheral eosinophilia > 10% of total WCC.
    - Peripheral neuropathy attributable to a systemic vasculitis.
    - Transient pulmonary infiltrates on chest X-ray (CXR).
    - Paranasal sinus abnormality.
    - Extravascular eosinophils seen on blood vessel biopsy.

11.8 GRANULOMATOSIS WITH POLYANGIITIS (GPA)

1. DEFINITION AND EPIDEMIOLOGY

- An ANCA-positive systemic vasculitis that involves small and medium-sized vessels with demonstration of presence of granulomas.
- Previously termed Wegener's granulomatosis.
- Prevalence of 160 cases per million.
    - Mean age of onset: $40 - 60$ years.
    - Caucasian population.
    - Incidence increases relative to distance from the equator.
    - No gender predominance.
- GPA can affect many organ systems, but the classical triad of involvement is:
    - Upper respiratory tract
    - Lower respiratory tract
    - Pauci-immune glomerulonephritis.

2. AETIOLOGY AND PATHOPHYSIOLOGY

- Aetiology of the disease is poorly understood, but an auto-immune non-infectious aetiology has been suggested.
- Necrotising vasculitis and granuloma formation are the classical histopathological findings in this disease.
    - There are few or no immune deposits in affected tissue.
    - T cells are involved in granuloma formation and maintenance.
    - B cells are also implicated.

3. CLASSIFICATION AND DIAGNOSIS

- There is no widely accepted formal classification of this disease.
- The American College of Rheumatologists used the following criteria for patients being enrolled into research studies:

Respiratory Medicine

- Nasal or oral inflammation (e.g. oral ulcers or bloody/inflammatory nasal discharge).
- Abnormal CXR identifying pulmonary nodules, infiltrates or cavities.
- Microscopic haematuria.
- Biopsy confirmation of granulomatous inflammation of an artery or perivascular region.
- > 80% of patients with GPA are associated with ANCA +ve serology, usually PR3-ANCA, 20% patients have alternative ANCA and 10% of patients are ANCA negative.
  - Utilisation of ANCA serology can be used to replace histological diagnosis if appropriate clinical history and radiology are supportive

11.9 MICROSCOPIC POLYANGIITIS (MPA)

- A poorly defined autoimmune disease characterised by necrotising small vessel vasculitis without evidence of granulomatous inflammation.
- Previously termed polyarteritis nodosa.
- Usually the disease is p-ANCA positive.
- Clinically and pathologically there is much overlap with GPA and MPA. The presentation is usually insidious, with constitutional symptoms such as fever, weight loss and fatigue.
- It can develop into a rapidly progressive vasculitis, which can affect the lungs with breathlessness, wheeze and haemoptysis. Necrotising crescentic glomerulonephritis is characteristic of MPA.

11.10 GOODPASTURE'S SYNDROME

1. DEFINITION AND EPIDEMIOLOGY

- Goodpasture's syndrome (GS) is characterised by anti-glomerular basement membrane antibodies (anti-GBM) deposition within affected organs.
  - Although vasculitis is present in some diagnoses of GS, it is not primarily a vasculitis: it is an autoimmune disease.
  - It is included in this section as it is an important differential in lung disease with a vasculitic picture.
  - It presents with a rapidly progressive glomerulonephritis with 30–40% of patients having pulmonary involvement (mainly haemorrhage).
- GS is rare, with an estimated incidence of 2 cases per million.
- 80% of cases occur in Caucasians, and there is a male predominance.
- There are 2 peaks of onset:
  - 20 – 30 years.
  - 60 – 70 years.

2. AETIOLOGY AND PATHOPHYSIOLOGY

- Patients with GS have an antibody (anti-GBM) to the alpha-3 chain of type IV collagen which is found in the lung and glomeruli of the kidney.
  - Identification of the antibody alongside the clinical picture is diagnostic.
- There may be a genetic association and many patients will have a history of smoking or hydrocarbon exposure.

11.11 CONNECTIVE TISSUE DISEASE AND LUNG VASCULITIS

1. SYSTEMIC LUPUS ERYTHEMATOSUS (SLE)

- SLE can affect almost any organ system, it is an auto-immune disorder with anti-phospholipid and anti-nuclear antibodies (ANA).
- This can lead to underlying vasculitis within the lung and diffuse pulmonary haemorrhages creating a picture similar to primary vasculitis.
- SLE can present as a pulmonary renal syndrome.
- It is more common in females, Afro-Caribbeans and younger patients.
- Skin and joint manifestations usually predominate.

2. OTHER CONNECTIVE TISSUE DISORDERS

- Other systemic disorders can affect the lung such as:
  - Rheumatoid arthritis
  - Systemic sclerosis
  - Ankylosing spondylitis.
- All of these disorders classically cause lung fibrosis, rather than a vasculitic picture and are therefore not discussed here (see Chapter 12: Interstitial lung disease).

11.12 PRESENTATION, INVESTIGATION AND MANAGEMENT OF VASCULITIS

1. PRESENTATION

- Vasculitis involving the lung can have a variety of signs and symptoms involving both the upper and lower respiratory tract, as well as systemic manifestations (See Figure 11.6).
- Specific symptoms are more typical of certain causes, as well as the speed of onset.

Respiratory Medicine

Respiratory symptoms

- **Upper respiratory symptoms (more typical of EGPA or GPA):**
  - Allergic rhinitis or sinusitis (in EGPA).
  - Nasal discharge.
  - Facial pain.
  - Oral and nasal ulcers.
  - Hoarseness.
  - Stridor.
  - Epistaxis.
  - Saddle-nose deformity (in EGPA).
- **Lower respiratory symptoms:**
  - Shortness of breath (SOB).
  - Cough.
  - Wheeze.
  - Tachypnoea.
  - History of asthma (in EGPA).
  - Haemoptysis.
  - Chest pain.

Extra-respiratory symptoms

- **Constitutional features:**
  - Fever (in GS).
- **Skin lesions:**
  - Pupura.
  - Petechiae.
  - Nodules.
  - Haemorrhage.
  - Ulcers.
- **Musculoskeletal:**
  - Myalgia.
  - Arthralgia.
  - Joint swelling.
  - Muscle weakness.
- **Neurological:**
  - Mononeuritismultiplex (in GPA or EGPA).
  - Focal numbness or weakness (in EGPA).
- **Renal:**
  - Decreased urinary output.

Figure 11.6 Clinical features of vasculitic diseases that affect the lung.

2. INVESTIGATIONS

- Investigation findings in vasculitis are listed in Table 11.2.

Table 11.2 **Investigations in suspected vasculitis of the lung.**

INVESTIGATIONS	FINDINGS
Full blood count (FBC)	Eosinophilia in EGPA, leukopenia in SLE.
Urea and electrolytes (U&E)	U&E may be deranged with a raised creatinine if the kidney is involved in any of the vasculitides.
Erythrocyte sedimentation rate (ESR) and C-reactive protein (CRP)	Will be raised in active disease with any of the vasculitides.
Urinalysis and microscopy	Haematuria and casts will be seen in EGPA, GS and SLE. MPA: proteinuria and haematuria.

(Continued)

Table 11.2 **(continued) Investigations in suspected vasculitis of the lung.**

INVESTIGATIONS	FINDINGS
ANCA, ANA, anti-GBM antibodies	EGPA: pANCA +ve. GPA: cANCA +ve. GS: anti-GBM +ve, ANCA: may be +ve. SLE: ANA +ve (anti-dsDNA and anti-Smith more specific). MPA: pANCA +ve.
Complement	Low levels of complement in SLE.
Clotting screen	Needed in suspected GS before performing renal biopsy. Prothrombin time (PT) will be prolonged in SLE.
Chest X-ray or computed tomography (CT)	Will show transient interstitial infiltrates or nodules in EGPA. GPA may show cavitating lung nodules and infiltrate. In GS there may be lung shadowing due to pulmonary haemorrhage.
Pulmonary function tests	Will show reversible airway obstruction in EGPA. Will show elevated diffusion capacity in pulmonary haemorrhage.
Renal biopsy	Will show crescentic glomerulonephritis, and characteristic linear IgG staining on immunofluorescence in GS.

3. MANAGEMENT

- Rapid diagnosis and treatment is critical to prevent death and long-term end organ damage.
- Management is usually done in conjunction with renal specialists and/or rheumatologists.
- Corticosteroids are the mainstay of treatment in all causes of lung vasculitis.
- Steroids are combined with other immunosuppressive agents used either to induce remission or to maintain disease control.
  - Examples include cyclophosphamide, azathioprine, mycophenolate and rituximab.
- Plasmapheresis is sometimes used in severe renal or pulmonary disease.
- Patients on long-term immunosuppression are usually offered *Pneumocystis jirovecii* prophylaxis:
  - Co-trimoxazole 150 mg once a day (OD).

4. PROGNOSIS

- The prognosis of vasculitic disease in the lung is dependent on the cause as well as the speed of treatment initiation.

Respiratory Medicine

- EGPA prognosis is highly dependent on extent and severity of organ involvement, but with appropriate immunosuppression survival is similar to age matched controls.
- GPA has a poor prognosis untreated with median survival of 5 months, but aggressive immunosuppression regimens achieve remission for most patients.
  - Morbidity in these patients is common as most will suffer long-term complications.
  - Almost half of patients will suffer a relapse in their lifetime.
- GS has a good prognosis with early aggressive treatment.
  - Over 90% of patients will recover and not require dialysis.
  - If dialysis is required on admission to hospital, the prognosis is much poorer as end-stage renal failure usually develops.

MICRO-case

A 30-year-old man presents with a 3-month history of nasal stuffiness, haemoptysis and epistaxis, associated with shortness of breath, weight loss and night sweats. Examination revealed crusting of his nares. Initial blood tests revealed elevated white cell count (neutrophilia) and anaemia. There is evidence of acute kidney injury on his U&E, with a urine dipstick positive for blood. CT chest demonstrates multiple infiltrative lesions and bronchoscopy shows evidence of recent haemorrhage with cytology demonstrating eosinophilia. As vasculitis is suspected, an ANCA screen is sent. The patient is positive for cANCA and anti-PR3, confirming granulomatosis with polyangiitis. He deteriorates rapidly, necessitating critical care input for type 1 respiratory failure and renal replacement therapy for acute kidney injury with oliguria. He is treated with high-dose glucocorticoids in combination with rituximab. Due to the severity of renal disease, he also undergoes plasma exchange. Following recovery from the acute episode, he continues on a reducing course of prednisolone, alongside rituximab. Co-trimoxazole is added for *P. jirovecii* prophylaxis and alendronic acid with calcium and vitamin D supplements for bone protection.

Key Points

- Granulomatosis with polyangiitis requires rapid diagnosis and treatment to prevent severe morbidity and mortality.
- Glucocorticoids in combination with other immunosuppressive agents (usually cyclophosphamide or rituximab) are the mainstay of treatment.
- An MDT approach is often necessary as patients may have extra-pulmonary manifestations (e.g. renal disease).
- Plasma exchange may be required in severe cases.
- Patients should receive prophylaxis against P. jirovecii when on high dose steroids.
- Vitamin D, calcium and bisphosphonates are given to protect against osteoporosis due to long-term steroid use.

Respiratory Medicine

Pulmonary Hypertension

12.1 PULMONARY HYPERTENSION

1. DEFINITION

- The 2022 European Society of Cardiology/European Respiratory Society (ESC/ERS) guidelines now define pulmonary hypertension (PH) by a mean pulmonary arterial pressure >20 mmHg at rest.
- The definition of pulmonary arterial hypertension (PAH) also implies a pulmonary vascular resistance (PVR) >2 Wood units and pulmonary arterial wedge pressure ≤15 mmHg.

2. CLASSIFICATION OF PH

- Patients are classified into World Health Organization (WHO) PH categories 1–5 (see Table 12.1).
  - Group 1 PH disorders are known as pulmonary arterial hypertension (PAH).
  - Groups 2–5 are referred to as PH but can also be used to refer to all five groups collectively.

Table 12.1 **WHO classification of PH.**

WHO PH GROUPS	WHO PH SUBGROUPS

Group 1: Pulmonary arterial hypertension (PAH)	**1. Idiopathic pulmonary arterial hypertension:**
	2. Heritable:
	  • BMRP2
	  • ALK 1, endolin
	  • Unknown
	3. Drug and toxin induced (e.g. dasatinib, dexfenfluramine, methamphetamines)
	4. Pulmonary arterial hypertension related to risk factors or associated conditions:
	  • Connective tissue disease
	  • HIV infection

(Continued)

DOI: 10.1201/9781315113937-13

Table 12.1 (*continued*) WHO classification of PH.

WHO PH GROUPS	WHO PH SUBGROUPS

	• Portal hypertension
	• Congenital heart disease
	• Schistosomiasis
	• Chronic haemolytic anaemia.
	5. **Pulmonary veno-occlusive disease and/or capillary haemangiotosis**
	6. **Pulmonary arterial hypertension related to risk factors or associated conditions:**
	  • Connective tissue disease
	  • HIV infection
	  • Portal hypertension
	  • Congenital heart disease
	  • Schistosomiasis
	  • Chronic haemolytic anaemia.

Group 2: Pulmonary hypertension due to left heart disease	1. **Systolic dysfunction** 2. **Diastolic dysfunction** 3. **Valvular disease.**
Group 3: Pulmonary hypertension due to lung disease/ hypoxia	1. **COPD.** 2. **Interstitial lung disease.** 3. **Other pulmonary disease with mixed restrictive and obstructive pattern.** 4. **Sleep disordered breathing.** 5. **Alveolar hypoventilation disorders.** 6. **Chronic exposure to high altitude.** 7. **Developmental abnormalities.**
Group 4: Chronic thromboembolic pulmonary hypertension (CTEPH)	
Group 5: Pulmonary hypertension with unclear/multifactorial mechanism	1. **Haematological disorders: myeloproliferative disorders, splenectomy.** 2. **Systemic disorders: sarcoidosis, Langerhans cell histiocytosis, lymphangioleiomyomatosis, neurofibromatosis, vasculitis.** 3. **Metabolic disorders: glycogen storage disease, Gaucher disease, thyroid disease.** 4. **Others: tumoral obstruction, fibrosing mediastinitis, chronic renal failure on dialysis.**

3. DIAGNOSIS OF PH

- Symptoms of PH are mainly linked to right ventricle (RV) dysfunction, and typically associated with dyspnoea on exercise in the earlier course of the disease. The cardinal symptom is dyspnoea on progressively minor exertion.
- Other common symptoms and clinical signs are listed in the section below.
- Identification of underlying diseases, especially left heart dysfunction and lung disease, as well as comorbidities, is essential to ensure proper classification, risk assessment, and treatment.
- The diagnostic approach requires a low threshold of suspicion of PH, echocardiographic confirmation and then fast-track referral to PH centres in patients with a high likelihood of PAH, CTEPH, or other forms of severe PH.

12.2 IDIOPATHIC PULMONARY ARTERIAL HYPERTENSION (IPAH)

1. DEFINITION

- IPAH is PAH in absence of identifiable cause, risk factors or family history.

2. EPIDEMIOLOGY

- IPAH is very rare with an incidence of 1–2 cases per million per year in Europe and America, and is 2–4 times more common in women than men.

3. PATHOPHYSIOLOGY

- Group 1 PAH is characterised by:
  - Proliferative vasculopathy of the small muscular pulmonary arterioles.
  - Medial hypertrophy.
  - Intimal hyperplasia.
  - Plexiform lesions:
    - A proliferation of endothelium and smooth muscle cells with accumulation of inflammatory cells.
    - They are a hallmark of IPAH but may also be seen in other forms of PH.
- Groups 2–5 have more heterogeneous changes but do share some features with Group 1 disease.
- Increased pulmonary resistance causes increased right heart afterload, which in turn leads to right heart failure.

Respiratory Medicine

MICRO-facts

PAH Diagnostic Criteria

- Right heart catheterisation is the gold standard for diagnosing and classifying PH.
- A mean pulmonary artery pressure ≥20 mmHg at rest confirms the presence of PH.
- A mean pulmonary wedge pressure <15 mmHg excludes PH due to left heart disease.
    - This is the pressure measured by wedging a pulmonary catheter with an inflated balloon into a small pulmonary arterial branch.
    - It provides an indirect measure of left atrial pressure.
- Chronic lung diseases and other causes of hypoxemia are mild or absent.
- Venous thromboembolic disease is absent.
- Absence of systemic disorders (e.g. sarcoidosis), haematological disorders (e.g. myeloproliferative diseases), and metabolic disorders (e.g. glycogen storage disease).

4. CLINICAL FEATURES

- **Symptoms:**
    - Shortness of breath on exertion.
    - Exertional syncope/presyncope.
    - Angina.
    - Palpitations.
    - Leg swelling.
- **Signs:**
    - Raised JVP with giant V waves.
    - Right ventricular heave.
    - Splitting of S2 with loud P2.
    - Tricuspid regurgitation murmur.
    - Hepatomegaly and exaggerated hepato-jugular reflux.
    - Ascites and peripheral oedema.
    - Cyanosis.

5. INVESTIGATIONS

- **Blood tests:**
    - Generally to rule out other causes of PH.
    - Autoantibodies to rule out connective tissue disease.
    - Thrombophilia screen.
    - Serum ACE.

- Thyroid function tests.
- HIV serology.

ECG:
- Signs of right ventricular hypertrophy.
- Right axis deviation.
- Dominant R wave in lead V1.
- P pulmonale.
- Incomplete RBBB.

CXR:
- Prominent pulmonary arteries.
- Cardiomegaly (See Figure 12.1).
- Pruning of peripheral lung vessels.

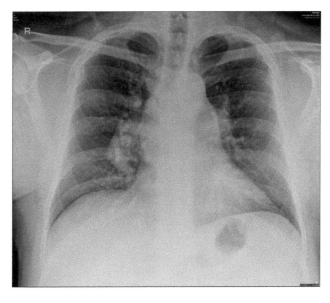

Figure 12.1 CXR of a patient with pulmonary hypertension showing prominent pulmonary arteries and cardiomegaly.

ECHO:
- Raised estimated systolic pulmonary artery pressure (>40 mmHg).
- Dilated right-sided chambers.
- Reduced right ventricular function.
- Right ventricular hypertrophy.
- Enlarged pulmonary artery.
- Paradoxical septal movement.

- **HRCT:**
  - Absence of underlying lung disease.
  - Centrilobular ground glass nodules can be evident.
- **CTPA/VQ scan:**
  - Assessment for presence of chronic thromboembolic disease (See Figure 12.2).

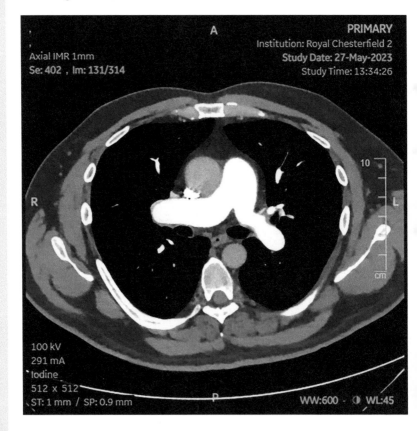

Figure 12.2 CTPA of a patient with pulmonary hypertension.

- **PFT:**
  - Mild restrictive or obstructive pattern in some patients.
  - Reduced T$_{LCO}$.
- **Abdominal ultrasound:**
  - Screen for portal hypertension.
- **Right heart catheter:**
  - Mean pulmonary artery pressure of more than 20 mmHg.
  - Pulmonary wedge pressure less than 15 mmHg.

- Normal or reduced cardiac output.
- Patients can also undergo vasodilator response test to assess likely response to calcium channel blockers during the procedure.

5. MANAGEMENT

- **General measures:**
  - Diuretics.
  - Oxygen therapy.
  - Oral anticoagulation (no clear guideline, must be individualised).
  - Influenza and pneumococcal vaccination.
  - Correction of anaemia.
- **Supportive therapy:**
  - Psychosocial support
  - Avoid excessive physical activity
  - Rehabilitation.
- **Vasoreactive response on right heart catheter:**
  - **Calcium channel blockers:**
    - Patients must be followed up to confirm they are long-term responders.
    - Examples include nifedipine and diltiazem.
- **Non-vasoreactive response on right heart catheter:**
  - **Prostacyclin analogues:**
    - Acts as a vasodilator and inhibits platelet aggregation.
    - Can be given as continuous IV infusion, subcutaneous infusion or nebulised.
    - Examples include epoprostenol and iloprost.
  - **Endothelin receptor antagonists:**
    - Counteracts vasoconstriction of vascular smooth muscle by endothelin.
    - Examples include bosentan and ambrisentan.
  - **Phosphodiesterase-5 inhibitors:**
    - Increases vasodilatory effects of nitric oxide.
    - Examples include sildenafil and tadalafil.
- **Balloon atrial septostomy:**
  - Atrial septostomy creates a right to left shunt within the atria.
  - This decompresses the right heart, increases left ventricular preload and improves cardiac output.
  - Can be used in patients awaiting transplantation, right heart failure refractory to medical therapy or with syncopal symptoms.
- **Transplantation:**
  - Indicated when there is inadequate response to other therapies especially in context of poor prognosis profile.
  - 5-year survival is 45 – 50%.

Respiratory Medicine

7. PROGNOSIS

- Prognosis is indicated by WHO functional classification (see Table 12.2).
  - Median survival of untreated patients with WHO functional class IV is 6 months.
  - Medial survival of untreated patients with WHO functional class III is 2.5 years.

Table 12.2 **WHO functional classification of PH.**

CLASS	WHO FUNCTIONAL CLASSIFICATION
I	Patients with pulmonary hypertension but without resulting limitations of physical activity. Ordinary physical activity does not cause undue fatigue or dyspnoea, chest pain, or heart syncope.
II	Patients with pulmonary hypertension resulting in slight limitation of physical activity. They are comfortable at rest. Ordinary physical activity results in undue fatigue or dyspnoea, chest pain, or heart syncope.
III	Patients with pulmonary hypertension resulting in marked limitation of physical activity. They are comfortable at rest. Less than ordinary physical activity causes undue fatigue or dyspnoea, chest pain, or heart syncope.
IV	Patients with pulmonary hypertension resulting in inability to carry on any physical activity without symptoms. These patients manifest signs of right heart failure. Dyspnoea and/or fatigue may be present even at rest. Discomfort is increased by physical activity.

Data from: Rich, S. Primary pulmonary hypertension: executive summary. Evian, France. World Health Organization, 1998.

MICRO-print
Indicators of poor prognosis in IPAH:

- Clinical evidence of right heart failure.
- Rapid progression of symptoms.
- Syncope.
- WHO functional class IV.
- 6-minute walk test of less than 300 m.
- Peak O2 consumption of cardio-pulmonary exercise test less than 12 mL/min/kg.
- Elevated or rising BNP levels.

12.3 PULMONARY HYPERTENSION DUE TO OTHER CAUSES

GROUP 2: PULMONARY HYPERTENSION DUE TO LEFT HEART DISEASE

This can be caused by systolic, diastolic or valvular dysfunction.

Passive backwards transmission of pressure increases pulmonary artery pressure.

Pulmonary vascular resistance is increased by increased vasomotor tone and structural remodelling in the pulmonary arteries.

Diagnosis is made on right heart catheterisation with the following criteria:
- Mean pulmonary arterial pressure ≥20 mmHg.
- Pulmonary wedge pressure ≥15 mmHg.
- Normal/reduced cardiac output.

Left atrial enlargement on echocardiogram is a useful marker for chronic left atrial hypertension.

Treatment should be aimed at the underlying heart disease. Drugs specific to the treatment of PAH are not recommended.

GROUP 3: PULMONARY HYPERTENSION DUE TO LUNG DISEASE AND/OR HYPOXIA

As this group covers a wide variety of causes, there are multiple factors in the development of PH including:
- Hypoxic vasoconstriction
- Mechanical stress from hyperinflation
- Loss of capillaries
- Inflammation
- Smoking.

PH is a poor prognostic factor in COPD and ILD.

Echo can be used to screen for PH but diagnosis should be confirmed with right heart catheter.

Management should be with treatment of the underlying lung disease and long-term oxygen therapy for hypoxic patients.

GROUP 4: CHRONIC THROMBOEMBOLIC PULMONARY HYPERTENSION (CTEPH)

Resolution of clot in PE occurs within 30 days in 90% of patients.

In CTEPH there is abnormal organisation of thromboemboli into endothelialised fibrotic lesions that cause either occlusion or stenosis of the vessels.

Peripheral vascular changes similar to those in IPAH occur in the peripheral vessels.

Respiratory Medicine

- Neovascularisation occurs via collateral vessels.
- Suspected cases should undergo V/Q scan. A normal scan rules out CTEPH
- Diagnosis is confirmed with right heart catheter.
- Patients should have lifelong anticoagulation and be referred for consideration of pulmonary endarterectomy or balloon pulmonary angioplasty.
- Medical therapies shown to reduce pulmonary vascular resistance and improve exercise capacity include oral riociguat, and subcutaneous treprostinil.

4. GROUP 5: PULMONARY HYPERTENSION WITH UNCLEAR/MULTIFACTORIAL MECHANISM

- This is a diverse group of patients who do not clearly fit into one of the other four WHO classifications.
- The causes of PH in this group include systemic diseases, haematological disorders and metabolic diseases.

MICRO-case

You are working as a respiratory physician in a district general hospital when a 60-year-old man is referred to you by one of your colleagues. The patient has noticed progressive shortness of breath over the last few months, and as part of his work-up, underwent an echocardiogram. He has been referred to yourself as his estimated pulmonary artery systolic pressure (PASP) in 60 mmHg. You note that there is no evidence of left heart disease on the echocardiogram but there is right ventricular hypertrophy.

An HRCT is performed to exclude any underlying disease (there is none) and a CTPA demonstrates no thromboembolic disease. There is no evidence of any underlying systemic disease on clinical assessment or blood tests.

You refer the patient for right heart catheterisation which confirms pulmonary arterial hypertension and demonstrates a pulmonary capillary wedge pressure <15 mmHg. The test also demonstrates a positive response to calcium channel blockers, so he is commenced on diltiazem.

Key Points

- The definitive diagnosis of PH requires right heart catheterisation, demonstrating a mean pulmonary artery pressure of >20 mmHg.
- To diagnose IPAH, other causes of pulmonary hypertension must be excluded.
- Individuals with IPAH may demonstrate a vasoactive response on right heart catheterisation, in which case calcium channel blockers are the mainstay of treatment.
- If there is no vasoactive response, then treatment is with prostacyclin analogues, endothelin receptor antagonists or phosphodiesterase-5 inhibitors.

13 Fungal Diseases of the Lung

13.1 ALLERGIC BRONCHOPULMONARY ASPERGILLOSIS (ABPA)

DEFINITION

- A chronic hypersensitivity reaction that occurs in response to an *Aspergillus* fungus, most commonly *Aspergillus fumigatus*.
- Diagnostic criteria:
  - History of asthma.
  - Positive skin prick test to *Aspergillus* antigen.
  - Elevated precipitating antibodies to *Aspergillus* species.
  - Elevated serum total IgE concentration >417 IU/mL (>1000 ng/mL).
  - Blood eosinophilia $> 500 / mm^3$.
  - Lung infiltrates on chest radiograph or chest high-resolution computed tomography (HRCT).
  - Central bronchiectasis on chest computed tomography (CT).
  - Elevated specific serum IgE and IgG to *A. fumigatus*.
- ABPA-S (seropositive) disease is defined by the first four criteria in the absence of central bronchiectasis.
- The minimal criteria to diagnose ABPA are:
  - History of asthma.
  - Immediate skin test reactivity to *A. fumigatus*.
  - Elevated serum total IgE.
  - Central bronchiectasis.
  - Elevated specific serum IgE and IgG to *A. fumigatus*.
- In CF the diagnosis can be more difficult. Proposed definition:
  - Deterioration in symptoms.
  - Serum IgE $> 1000 iu / ml$.

DOI: 10.1201/9781315113937-14

- Immediate skin prick test positivity to Aspergillus or elevated specific IgE to *Aspergillus*.
- IgG *Aspergillus* or precipitating antibodies.
- New chest radiology changes.

2. EPIDEMIOLOGY

- Patients usually have a history of asthma or cystic fibrosis (CF).
  - The disease is estimated to affect around 2% of asthmatics and up to 15% of those with CF.

3. AETIOLOGY AND RISK FACTORS

- Atopy is an important risk factor for developing ABPA.

4. PATHOPHYSIOLOGY

- The true mechanisms are not clearly understood.
- *Aspergillus fumigatus* colonises the bronchi. Airborne spores reach the alveoli where they germinate leading to inflammation caused by IgE- and IgG-mediated reactions.
- Underlying airway disease such as asthma or CF causes mucus hypersecretio and impairs mucociliary clearance.
  - This leads to increased trapping of spores and decreased clearance.
  - Increased germination of spores within the lung induces an immune response.
  - The proximal bronchi become dilated and filled with mucus plugs containing eosinophils and fungal hyphae.
  - Bronchial obstruction, inflammation and mucoid impaction can lead t fibrosis and respiratory compromise.

MICRO-print

Chronic aspergillosis can lead to complications:

- Chronic cavitary aspergillosis – cavities form in the lung without the presence of aspergilloma.
- Chronic fibrosing pulmonary aspergillosis – if aspergillosis remains untreated, it causes scarring of the lung tissue that is irreversible.

5. CLINICAL FEATURES

- Almost exclusively in those with a history of asthma or CF.
- Typically presents from teenage years until the fourth decade.
- Symptoms:
    - History of atopy
    - Cough
    - Wheeze
    - Purulent mucus production
    - Pleuritic chest pain.
- Signs:
    - Fever
    - Finger clubbing
    - Weight loss
    - Cyanosis (late feature).

6. INVESTIGATIONS

- Investigation findings in ABPI are listed in Table 13.1.

Table 13.1 **Investigations in patients with suspected ABPI.**

INVESTIGATIONS	RESULT
Aspergillus fumigatus skin test	Can be used as an initial screening test. Positive wheal and flare reaction (not specific). Further serological and radiographic tests are needed, so often excluded in favour of serology.
Serum total IgE	IgE > 400 IU/mL if skin prick test not positive, is highly suggestive of ABPA.
Specific IgE to *Aspergillus*	IgE RAST positivity evident.
Full blood count (FBC)	Peripheral blood eosinophilia.
Sputum culture and microscopy	Macroscopic mucus plugs may be expectorated. *A. fumigatus* may be cultured and eosinophils seen on microscopy. These findings, however, are non-specific.
Chest X-ray	Flitting consolidation due to mucus plugging can be seen +/– bronchiectatic change.
Chest computed tomography (CT)	CT describes central proximal bronchiectasis (see Figure 13.1).

Respiratory Medicine

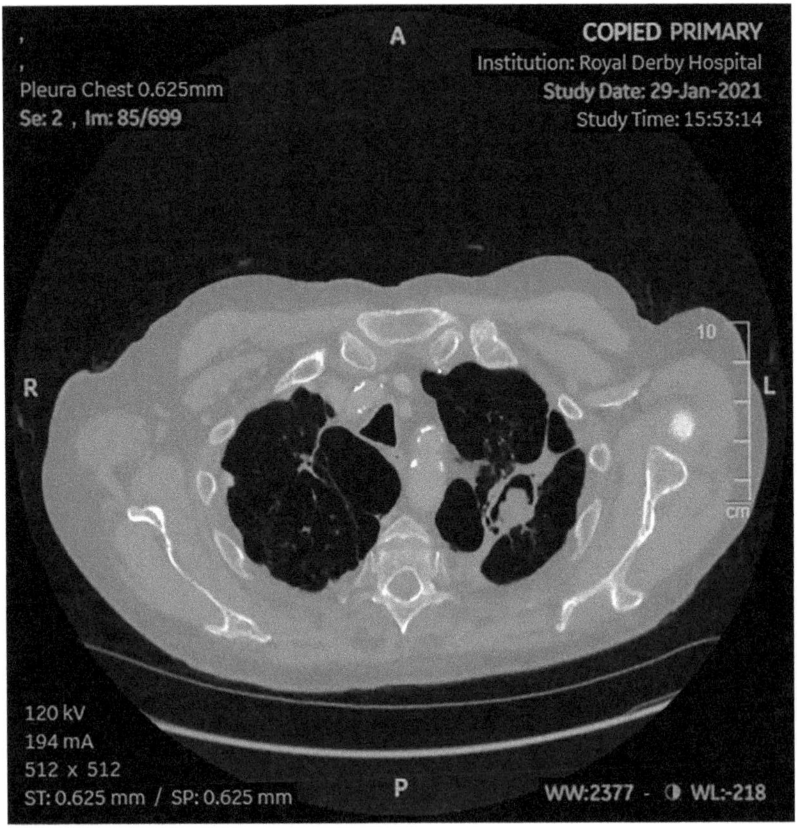

Figure 13.1 Chest CT of a patient with ABPA; the CT shows bilateral bronchiectasis and an aspergilloma in the left lung.

- Diagnosis of ABPI is separated clinically into 5 stages (see Micro-Facts box).

MICRO-facts

Stages of allergic bronchopulmonary aspergillosis (they are not necessarily consecutive):

Stage 1: acute

- Fever, cough, chest pain, haemoptysis, sputum.
- Infiltrates on CXR: upper or middle lobe.
- Serum IgE: markedly elevated.

Stage 2: remission

- Asymptomatic/stable asthma.

- No infiltrates on CXR when patient off prednisolone >6 months.
- Serum IgE: elevated or normal.

Stage 3: exacerbation

- Symptoms mimicking acute stage, or asymptomatic.
- Infiltrates on CXR: upper or middle lobe.
- Serum IgE: markedly elevated.

Stage 4: corticosteroid-dependent asthma

- Persistent severe asthma.
- Infiltrates on CXR: absent or only intermittent.
- Serum IgE: elevated or normal.

Stage 5: end-stage fibrosis

- Cyanosis and dyspnoea.
- Fibrotic, bullous, or cavitating lesions on CXR.

7. MANAGEMENT

- Prednisolone commenced at 30–40 mg with tapering over 3–6 months.
- Prolonged corticosteroid therapy will require bone protection, e.g. bisphosphonates.
- Itraconazole $200mg$ can be used as a steroid sparing agent:
  - Eliminates potential risk of adrenal suppression.
  - Affects the cytochrome $P450\ 3A4$ pathway.
  - Metabolism of inhaled budesonide and fluticasone can be reduced and so dose should be reduced.

MICRO-facts

Chronic pulmonary aspergillosis consists of five current consensus definitions:

- Chronic cavitatory pulmonary aspergillosis (CCPA) is the most common form: defined by one or more cavities, with or without a fungal ball present.
- Simple aspergilloma: Single fungal ball growing in a cavity.
- Aspergillus nodules: An unusual form of CPA, non-cavity forming, mimicking carcinoma of the lung or metastases and can only be definitively diagnosed using histology.
- Chronic fibrosing pulmonary aspergillosis (CFPA): Late-stage CCPA.
- Subacute invasive aspergillosis (SAIA) is very similar to CCPA but occurs in mildly immunocompromised or debilitated patients (e.g. diabetes mellitus, malnutrition, alcoholism, advanced age, prolonged steroid administration, COPD). Histology can often show tissue invasion. Progression is more rapid than with CCPA.

Respiratory Medicine

13.2 ASPERGILLOMA

1. DEFINITION

- A fungal mass that grows within a previous lung cavity.
- Most commonly an *Aspergillus* species causing an aspergilloma (otherwise termed a mycetoma).

2. RISK FACTORS

- Previous cavities formed within the lung are the main risk factor. Most of these are caused by:
  - Lung abscess
  - Lung cancer
  - Cystic fibrosis
  - Sarcoidosis
  - Tuberculosis
  - Bullous emphysema.

3. CLINICAL FEATURES

- Patients with mycetoma may be asymptomatic for decades until the disease becomes advanced.
  - May be found incidentally on chest X-ray or CT scan and potentially mimic lung cancer.
- Symptoms:
  - Cough.
  - Haemoptysis (rarely can cause life-threatening haemorrhage).
- Diagnosis.
- Soft tissue mass within an air-filled cavity visible on chest X-ray and CT (See Figure 13.2).
- IgG to *Aspergillus*/aspergillus precipitins may be raised.

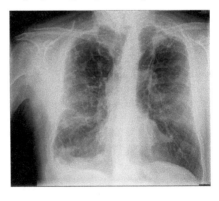

Figure 13.2 CXR of a patient with ABPA and aspergillomas, mucus plugging and bronchiectatic changes can be seen with multiple air-filled cavities.

4. MANAGEMENT

- Asymptomatic mycetomas do not require treatment.
  - There is poor evidence for the effectiveness of antifungal drugs.
- Adequate treatment of underlying disease, such as TB, is effective at preventing their occurrence.
- Rarely, surgical removal may be needed due to complications secondary to the mycetoma:
  - Major haemorrhage
  - Pleural empyema
  - Pneumothorax.
- Bronchial artery embolisation can be considered if there is persistent haemoptysis.

13.3 CHRONIC CAVITARY PULMONARY ASPERGILLOSIS (CCPA)

1. DEFINITION

- Expansion of pulmonary cavity due to aspergillus on imaging.
- Elevated aspergillus precipitins.
- Usually in immunocompetent patients.

2. RISK FACTORS

- Pre-existing pulmonary cavity
- Chronic lung disease
- Oral steroid use.

3. CLINICAL FEATURES

- Weight loss
- Breathlessness
- Cough
- Haemoptysis
- Fatigue.

4. INVESTIGATIONS

Radiology:

- Evolving and expanding cavities over months on either serial CXR or CT.
- Mycetoma may not be visible.
- Fibrosis can develop (late-stage complication known as chronic fibrosing aspergillosis).

Respiratory Medicine

Microbiology:

- Culture sputum for fungi, bacteria and atypical mycobacterial infection (can be co-existent).
- Negative culture for aspergillus does not exclude chronic cavitatory/fibrosis aspergillosis.

Serology:

- Serum IgG *Aspergillus* should be raised.
- Serum beta D-glucan can be raised.
- Serum galactomannan usually negative.
- Raised inflammatory markers (white cell count, C-reactive protein and erythrocyte sedimentation rate) can be seen.

5. MANAGEMENT

- Rule out intercurrent bacterial and mycobacterial infection.
- Antifungals if clinical symptoms and radiology is evolving.
- Use either itraconazole, voriconazole, posaconazole.
- Careful monitoring is required if on antifungal treatment including monitoring of liver function tests (risk of hepatoxicity with antifungals).
- Treatment response guided by improvement in symptoms, stabilising of radiology and improvement in aspergillus serology and inflammatory markers.

13.4 SUBACUTE INVASIVE ASPERGILLOSIS (SAIA)

1. DEFINITION

- Aspergillus invasion of tissue in patients with risk factors for immunosuppression with raised aspergillus serology.
- Cavitating pneumonia or thin-walled cavity on chest radiology.

2. RISK FACTORS

- COPD.
- Chronic high use of alcohol.
- Diabetes mellitus.
- Poor nutrition/low body mass index.
- Frequent or long-term oral steroid use.
- Immunosuppressive treatment.
- Older age.

3. CLINICAL FEATURES

- Similar to chronic cavitatory aspergillosis.
- Evolution of clinical symptoms and radiology is between 1 and 3 months.

Respiratory Medicine

4. INVESTIGATIONS

Radiology

- Usually upper zone changes/opacification on initial imaging.
- Air crescent sign on CT in early stage.
- Cavity develops +/– mycetoma with time.
- In later stages, multiple cavities with adjacent pleural involvement.

Microbiology

- Culture sputum for fungi, bacteria and atypical mycobacterial infection.
- Ideally have tissue biopsy to demonstrate.

Serology

- Serum IgG *Aspergillus* likely to be raised.
- Serum galactomannan can be positive.

5. MANAGEMENT

- Similar to management of chronic cavitatory aspergillosis except narrower spectrum of antifungals to choose from.
- Antifungal of choice is voriconazole.

13.5 INVASIVE ASPERGILLOSIS

1. DEFINITION

- Inhalation of Aspergillus spores leads to colonisation of the individual. It is defined as invasive aspergillosis when tissue invasion occurs.
  - Defective immunity then predisposes to tissue invasion.

2. EPIDEMIOLOGY

- Patient groups affected by invasive aspergillosis are shown in Figure 13.3.

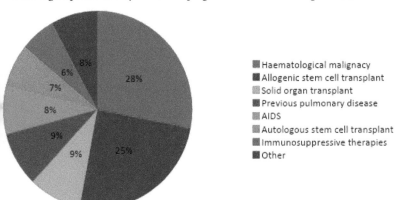

- Haematological malignacy
- Allogenic stem cell transplant
- Solid organ transplant
- Previous pulmonary disease
- AIDS
- Autologous stem cell transplant
- Immunosuppressive therapies
- Other

Figure 13.3 Patient groups affected by invasive aspergillosis.

Respiratory Medicine

3. AETIOLOGY

- *Aspergillus fumigatus* is the most common pathogenic species causing up to 70% of disease.
- Other pathogens that cause invasive aspergillosis:
  - *Aspergillus flavus.*
  - *Aspergillus terreus.*
  - *Aspergillus niger.*

4. PATHOPHYSIOLOGY

- Aerosolised spores (conidia) of the *Aspergillus* species are inhaled and colonise the bronchi.
- If the conidia survive, they germinate into filamentous hyphae, which invades the pulmonary parenchyma.
- Neutropenia and defective T-lymphocyte function predispose to tissue invasion.
- The hyphae become angio-invasive and gain entry to the pulmonary microvasculature.
- Thrombi with inflammation and pulmonary infarction develop, which consequently causes the symptomology.
- Widespread dissemination can occur through haematological spread. Most commonly travelling to the brain and skin.

5. CLINICAL FEATURES

- Symptoms:
  - Pleuritic chest pain
  - Cough
  - Haemoptysis
  - Headache
  - Dyspnoea
  - Congestion
  - Sinus tenderness or facial pain
  - Seizures.
- Signs:
  - Nasal ulcers
  - Skin rash
  - Fever
  - Weight loss
  - Altered mental status
  - Weight loss.

INVESTIGATIONS

Investigation findings in invasive aspergillosis are listed in Table 13.2.

Table 13.2 **Investigations in suspected invasive aspergillosis.**

INVESTIGA-TIONS	RESULT
Chest X-ray (CXR)	May show nodules, consolidation, infiltrates, cavities and pleural lesions. Sometimes the CXR is normal.
High-resolution CT (HRCT)	**Chest:** The pathognomonic sign are nodules (usually >1 cm) with a halo or air crescent. These may not be present consistently. Other non-specific signs are ground glass opacity, micronodules, infiltrates, pleural effusion, pleural thickening, aspergilloma, upper lobe cavity mass. **Respiratory sinuses:** mass within the sinus cavity and bone erosions of the sinus wall **Brain:** focal lesions.
MRI head	Space occupying lesions or abscesses, with surrounding oedema and haemorrhage. A mass and bony erosion may be seen within the sinuses.
Serum galactomannan enzyme immunoassay (EIA)	A positive EIA for galactomannan antigen (constituent of polysaccharide wall of *Aspergillus* and some other fungi) on a serum sample is highly sensitive and specific. In a high-risk patient with positive radiological findings, a positive result can remove the need for invasive diagnostic procedures.
BAL galactomannan	Detection can reflect potentially invasive disease and may be more sensitive compared to culture. False positive testing can occur.
Serum beta-D-glucan	1,3 beta-D-glucan is a constituent of fungal walls including *Aspergillus* and PCP (see below). Detection can reflect IA but also other fungal infections.
Sputum smear and culture	Sputum is usually absent in patients with aspergillosis. If present, smear and culture may be done: this may show hyphae on a smear and *Aspergillus* species on culture. Interpretation of this is problematic and dependent on whether the patient is immunodeficient.
Tissue biopsy, culture and staining	Gold standard for diagnosis. Video-assisted thoracoscopic (VATS) biopsy is the preferred method. Biopsy may show septate hyphae with angioinvasion, inflammation and tissue necrosis as well as aspergilloma, fungal mycelia, fibrin, mucus and tissue debris. Culture may confirm an *Aspergillus* species.

Respiratory Medicine

7. DIFFERENTIAL DIAGNOSIS

- Fungal differentials:
  - Mucormycosis:
    - Infection by fungi in the order Mucorales.
    - Brain, respiratory sinus and lungs are most commonly affected.
  - Fusariosis:
    - Infection by fungus of Fusarium species, usually in immunocompromised neutropenic patients.
  - Scedosporiosis:
    - Infection by fungus in Scedosporium genus.
    - Resistant to antifungals with a very poor prognosis.
- Non-fungal differentials:
  - Cavitating infarction due to PE.
  - Malignancy.
  - Mycobacterial infection.
  - Pneumonia.
  - Nocardiosis.

8. MANAGEMENT

- To successfully treat IA, it is essential that:
  - The underlying immune deficiency in the patient is reversed.
  - Antifungal therapy is started early: this may be preemptive, empiric or definitive. The following antifungals can be used:
    - Azoles (e.g. voriconazole, posaconazole)
    - Polyenes (e.g. amphotericin B).
    - Echinocandins (e.g. caspofungin, micafungin).
  - The flowchart below (Figure 13.4) summarises the treatment algorithm used for invasive aspergillosis.

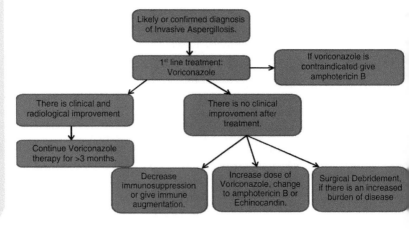

Figure 13.4 Treatment algorithm for invasive aspergillosis.

9. COMPLICATIONS

- Haemoptysis: often can be massive and life-threatening.
- Disseminated disease:
    - Can affect all organ systems, with a mortality of almost 90%.
- Obstructive pneumonia.
- Severe hypoxia.
- Pericarditis.

10. PROGNOSIS

- Successful outcomes are dependant on:
    - Early diagnosis and anti-fungal initiation.
    - Successful treatment of underlying immunodeficiency.
- Risk of death is higher in patients that have:
    - Severe underlying disease.
    - Large lesions or a high number of them on CXR.
    - A high *Aspergillus* IgG titre.
    - Continuing immunosuppression.

13.6 PNEUMOCYSTIS PNEUMONIA (PCP/PJP)

1. DEFINITION

- PCP is an opportunistic infection of the lung, caused by the fungal organism **Pneumocystis jirovecii** (formerly **Pneumocystis carinii**).
    - It normally only causes disease in the immunocompromised; disease in immunocompetent individuals has been described but is extremely rare.
    - It is one of the AIDS-defining illnesses.

2. EPIDEMIOLOGY

- HIV +ve patients are the most common group in which PCP occurs.
    - Almost exclusively within patients with a CD4 count < 200 cells/microliter.
- The other patient groups in which PCP occurs are patients with:
    - Solid organ transplant.
    - Haematological malignancy.
    - Inflammatory conditions requiring immunosuppression.

3. AETIOLOGY

- **P. jirovecii** is commonly found in the lungs of healthy individuals.
    - Pathogen spread is via airborne transmission.
    - It only causes disease when both cellular and humoral immunity are defective.

4. PATHOPHYSIOLOGY

- The pathophysiology of PCP infection is shown as a flowchart in Figure 13.5

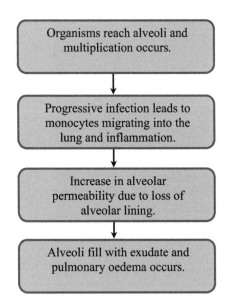

Figure 13.5 Pathophysiology of PCP infection.

5. CLINICAL FEATURES

- Symptoms:
    - Dyspnoea, especially on exercise.
    - Cough:
        - Usually non-productive.
        - Haemoptysis (rare).
    - Fever.
    - Chest pain.
    - Weight loss.
- Signs:
    - Tachycardia.
    - Fever.
    - Tachypnoea.
    - Dramatic desaturations on exercise on a background of normal saturations.
    - Cyanosis (rare).

- Chest signs:
  - Crackles
  - Bronchial breathing
  - Often normal.

MICRO-print

Rarely *Pneumocystis* infections can cause extra-pulmonary manifestations. This is usually in patients with advanced HIV infection not taking prophylaxis. This can occur without any pulmonary involvement. It may present in the following systems:

- Eyes
- Lymphadenopathy
- Thyroid
- GI tract
- Bone marrow
- Central nervous system.

---

6. INVESTIGATIONS

- The investigation of PCP infection is summarised in Table 13.3.

Table 13.3 **Investigations in possible PCP.**

INVESTIGATIONS	RESULT
Chest X-ray (CXR)	Bilateral perihilar opacities are typical; these may be reticular or granular. The CXR may have a variety of appearances e.g. there may be pneumatoceles or cysts (See Figure 13.6).
Induced sputum	Induced sputum can be sent for staining for *P. jirovecii* to confirm the diagnosis. Direct fluorescent antigen testing or PCR can be done on the sputum sample which has excellent sensitivity and specificity if the sputum sample is of adequate quality
Serum LDH	LDH levels are increased in 90% of HIV patients infected with PCP. This can be used to monitor therapy: it should decline with successful treatment.
High resolution computed tomography (HRCT)	Ground glass opacities can be seen in addition to septal thickening and pneumatoceles.
Bronchoalveolar lavage (BAL)	BAL can be done if the induced sputum is negative as it has a higher diagnostic yield.

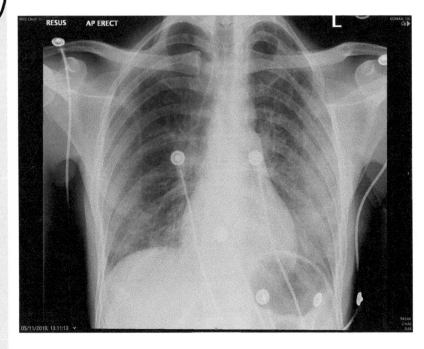

Figure 13.6 Chest CT of patient with PCP; the CT shows septal thickening and ground glass changes.

7. DIFFERENTIAL DIAGNOSIS

- There are many respiratory diseases with similar presentations to PCP:
  - Infectious:
    - Bacterial pneumonia
    - Viral pneumonia
    - Influenza
    - Pulmonary TB
    - Mycobacterium avium complex (MAC)
    - Cytomegalovirus (CMV)
    - Coccidioidomycosis
    - Histoplasmosis
    - Cryptococcus
    - Blastomycosis
    - Penicillinosis.
  - Non-infectious:
    - Acute respiratory distress syndrome (ARDS)
    - Lymphocytic interstitial pneumonia

- Sarcoidosis
- Kaposi sarcoma
- Interstitial lung disease.

8. MANAGEMENT

- The first-line treatment for PCP is co-trimoxazole $15 - 20mg / kg$ /day (trimethoprim/sulfamethoxazole).
  - Treatment course is typically for 3 weeks.
- In severe PCP infection the patient may need:
  - Mechanical ventilation.
  - Prednisolone 40 mg PO BD (with a reducing regime after 5 days of therapy).

9. COMPLICATIONS

- Complications that occur with PCP may be due to the disease itself or drugs used to treat it:
  - Respiratory failure.
  - ARDS.
  - Pneumothorax.
  - Immune-reconstitution inflammatory syndrome (IRIS).
    - In AIDS patients due to restoration of immune function on highly active antiretroviral therapy (HAART).
  - Drug adverse reactions including kidney injury.
  - Death.

10. PROGNOSIS

- Mortality for PCP is around 11% the following factors increase the chance of a poor prognosis:
  - Increasing patient age
  - Medical co-morbidities
  - Previous PCP episodes
  - Pulmonary Kaposi sarcoma
  - AIDS diagnosis (CD4 count < 200)
  - Being HIV negative
  - Illicit drug use.
- Clinical indicators of a poor prognosis:
  - Increased respiratory rate.
  - Decreased partial pressure of O_2 on room air.
  - Hypoalbuminaemia.
  - ↑ White cell count.
  - ↓ Haemoglobin on admission.
  - Neurological signs and symptoms.
  - Patient requiring mechanical ventilation.

Respiratory Medicine

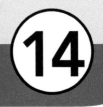

Sleep Disordered Breathing

14.1 OBSTRUCTIVE SLEEP APNOEA/ HYPOPNOEA SYNDROME (OSAHS)

1. DEFINITION

- OSAHS is a sleep disordered breathing syndrome characterised by episodes of partial or complete upper airway collapse during sleep causing significant daytime sleepiness.
- An apnoea is a 10-second or greater pause in breathing.
- Hypopnoea is a 10-second or greater reduction in airflow by at least 30% with oxygen desaturation of 3%.
- Apnoea/hypopnoea index (AHI): number of apnoeic and hypopnoeic events per hour.

2. EPIDEMIOLOGY

- OSAHS is a common and under-diagnosed condition with a prevalence of 4% in men and 2% in women.
- Prevalence is related to levels of obesity.

3. AETIOLOGY

- Structural causes:
  - Craniofacial abnormalities.
  - Mandibular hypoplasia or retroposition.
  - Nasal obstruction from causes such as polyps and septal deviation.
  - Macroglossia.
  - Adenotonsillar hypertrophy.
  - Pharyngeal fat deposition.
- Non-structural risk factors:
  - Male sex.
  - Obesity.
  - Increasing age.
  - Use of sedatives or alcohol.

DOI: 10.1201/9781315113937-15

- Smoking.
- Family history.

4. PATHOPHYSIOLOGY

- Airway collapse secondary to pharyngeal dilator muscles inability to maintain patency due to muscle relaxation/weakness and/or small pharyngeal size.
- The patient may undergo apnoea or hypopnoea associated with hypoxia and possibly hypercapnia resulting in arousal.
  - The patient is not aware of this, but it is detectable on EEG (electroencephalogram) and results in fragmented sleep and daytime somnolence.
- Arousal is associated with increased blood pressure, up to an increase of 50 mmHg.
  - Effective treatment of OSAHS with CPAP (continuous positive airway pressure) reduces daytime blood pressure by 3 mmHg.
  - The rise in blood pressure is also associated with a rise in pulse.
- Hypoxia causes oxidative stress, which along with the cardiovascular disruption of OSAHS is thought to contribute to:
  - Atherosclerosis
  - Myocardial ischaemia
  - Left ventricular hypertrophy
  - Left ventricular failure
  - Cardiac arrhythmias
  - Cerebrovascular disease
  - Metabolic syndrome
  - Insulin resistance.

MICRO-facts

Taking a sleep history:
- Quality of sleep.
- Quantity of sleep.
- Shift work.
- Use of sedatives.
- Use of alcohol.
- Unusual behaviour during sleep.
- Signs of restless leg syndrome.
- Signs of depression.

5. CLINICAL FEATURES

- The most common presentation is excessive daytime somnolence and unrefreshing sleep.
- A collateral history may identify snoring or apnoeic episodes unknown to the patient.

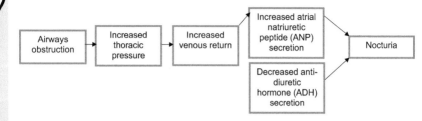

Figure 14.1 Pathophysiology of nocturia in OSAHS.

- Patient may report waking up choking.
- Irritability, change in personality or poor concentration.
- Morning headache reflects significant nocturnal hypoventilation.
- Decreased libido/impotence.
- Nocturia (see Figure 14.1).
- Occupation: daytime somnolence may impact upon driving.
  - Occupation may be relevant, e.g. HGV drivers may be unsafe to continue with driving if OSAHS is untreated.
- There are many causes of disturbed sleep and sleepiness so a full sleep history must be obtained (see MICRO-Facts box).

6. EXAMINATION

- Record weight and BMI.
- Neck circumference more than 17 inches is associated with OSAHS.
- Inspect mandibular size, teeth and oropharynx for crowding, enlarged tonsils and macroglossia.
- Assess nasal patency.
- In addition, examine for signs or respiratory or cardiovascular disease.

7. INVESTIGATIONS

- Epworth Sleepiness Scale (ESS), available at https://epworthsleepinessscale.com:
  - A subjective measure of how likely a patient is to fall asleep in a given circumstance.
  - A score of more than 10 is considered clinically relevant.
  - This can be completed both by the patient, and by relative or partner, as the patient may underestimate their symptoms.
  - ESS of more than 10 with symptoms of OSAHS, or sleepiness in dangerous conditions with normal ESS but in presence of symptoms of OSAHS should prompt referral for investigation.
- Overnight oximetry
  - Pulse oximetry can be used as a first line screening tool for OSAHS.

- A finger or earlobe pulse oximeter records heart rate and oxygen saturations overnight. Oxygen desaturation index (ODI) reflects the number of desaturation episodes >4% per hour.
- Interpretation of oximetry by an experienced practitioner can diagnose OSAHS, but a normal tracing does not exclude the diagnosis.
- Limited sleep studies
  - A limited sleep study may measure pulse oximetry, thoraco-abdominal movement, nasal airflow snoring, heart rate, and body movement.
  - Limited sleep studies can be performed at home after instruction from a sleep technician.
  - Limited sleep studies are adequate for diagnosis of OSAHS in the majority of patients.
- Polysomnography (PSG):
  - To perform PSG the patient must attend a sleep centre for overnight monitoring with EEG, electromyogram (EMG), electro-oculogram, oronasal flow monitors, thoraco-abdominal movement and oximetry tracing.
  - Although PSG has been considered the gold standard for diagnosing OSAHS, it is expensive and time-consuming.
  - Overnight hospital PSG is appropriate for a small number of patients who cannot be investigated at home, or whose home study does not fit with the clinical picture.

MICRO-facts

Assessment of severity of OSAHS:
- **Mild:** AHI 5–14/hr.
- **Moderate:** AHI 15–30/hr.
- **Severe:** >30/hr.

3. MANAGEMENT

- Conservative management:
  - Weight loss should be encouraged with or without CPAP.
  - Patients should avoid alcohol in the evening, and minimise the use of sedatives or sleeping tablets.
  - The patient should avoid sleeping on their back if non-sleepy snorers.
- Continuous positive airway pressure (CPAP):
  - Splints the upper airway preventing collapse, and therefore sleep fragmentation.
  - Indicated in symptomatic moderate and severe OSAHS. There is no evidence for use in mild OSAHS.

Respiratory Medicine

- CPAP improves objective and subjective sleepiness, cognitive function, mood, blood pressure and quality of life.
- Requires an adjustment period with input from a sleep technician to maximise compliance and time on machine.
- Common side effects include rhinitis, pressure sores from mask, discomfort, claustrophobia, abdominal bloating and noise, but intensive input from a sleep technician can minimise these.
- Mandibular advancement device (MAD):
  - MADs work by producing anterior displacement of the mandible increasing upper airway diameter.
  - Fits to the upper and lower teeth, and allows the lower jaw to be displaced forward by $5-10mm$.
  - MADs are suitable in mild OSAHS and excessive snoring, and can be tried in patients unable to tolerate CPAP.
- Surgical management:
  - There is no evidence supporting the use of surgical techniques such as uvulopalatopharyngoplasty or mandibular advancement osteotomy for the treatment of snoring or OSAHS.

MICRO-print
Driving Advice

- All patients should be advised not to drive when sleepy and advised that falling asleep at the wheel is a criminal offence.
- When diagnosed, patients should be told to inform the DVLA of the diagnosis. They will also need to inform their insurance company.
- If the patient is symptomatic, then they should not drive. Once their symptoms are controlled and have been reviewed, they can resume driving.
- Holders of a bus, coach or lorry licence cannot resume driving until they have been reviewed in a specialist clinic, have a normal ESS and have adequate usage of their CPAP machine.
- www.gov.uk/excessive-sleepiness-and-driving

14.2 CENTRAL SLEEP APNOEA

- Central sleep apnoea is defined by reduction or absence of ventilation lasting more than 10 seconds due to loss of neural output to the respiratory muscles.
- Cheyne-Stokes respiration refers to periods of hyperventilation alternating with central apnoea.
- It is associated with heart failure, PH, stroke, neuromuscular disease, obesity hypoventilation syndrome and drug use.
- CPAP, Adapto-Servo ventilation or BiPAP can be used to manage this condition.

14.3 SLEEP-RELATED HYPOVENTILATION

- Sleep-related hypoventilation is defined as an increased $pCO2 > 6kPA$ during sleep, or disproportionately raised nocturnal $pCO2$ compared to daytime levels.
- Sleep-related hypoventilation can be caused by decreased ventilatory drive, or by failure of the mechanical aspect of ventilation.
- Obesity hypoventilation disorder (previously called Pickwickian syndrome) is the association of obesity and alveolar hypoventilation leading to hypercapnia. Respiratory failure is present in the awake daytime state. Often overlaps with OSAHS with similar symptoms.

14.4 OTHER CAUSES OF POOR SLEEP/ DAYTIME SOMNOLENCE

- Shift work patterns
- High caffeine intake
- Alcohol intake
- Drugs, e.g. benzodiazepines
- Nocturia
- Restless legs syndrome.

Respiratory Medicine

15

Occupational Lung Disease

15.1 WORK-RELATED ASTHMA

1. DEFINITION

- Work-related asthma (WRA) is subdivided into three main phenotypes:
    - Work-aggravated asthma (WAA).
    - Allergic occupational asthma due to allergic sensitisation.
    - Irritant-induced asthma (IIA).
- Patients with WAA either have pre-existing asthma or develop coincidental adult-onset asthma and report symptoms that are made worse by non-specifi factors in the workplace such as exercise, cold air or dust.
- In contrast, occupational asthma is caused by airborne exposures in the working environment.

2. EPIDEMIOLOGY

- Occupational asthma accounts for 1 in 6 cases of adult asthma.
- The reported incidence of occupational asthma is between 12 and 300 cases million workers/year.
    - The true incidence is likely to be higher as it is an under-diagnosed disease.
- One-third of patients diagnosed with occupational asthma are unemployed up to 6 years after diagnosis.

3. AETIOLOGY

- Inhaled aeroallergens can cause symptoms via immunological or non-immunological means.
- **Immunologically mediated occupational asthma:**
    - Repeated exposure to high-molecular-weight agents and some low-molecular-weight agents triggers an IgE response to the inhaled substance.
        - These sensitiser-induced cases have a latency period between exposure to the sensitiser and development of asthma symptoms.

DOI: 10.1201/9781315113937-16

- In some patients with disease caused by low-molecular-weight agents, there is often no clear IgE antigen detectable, or only detectable in some.
  - Patients in this group have symptoms consistent with allergic disease and have reproducible symptoms to specific challenge tests.
  - This subgroup of patients tend to be non-atopic non-smokers, and have atypical or late asthmatic reactions.
- **Non-immunological occupational asthma:**
  - There is no latency period between expose and symptoms.
  - The symptoms are provoked by exposure to a high concentration of irritant agent.

4. SYMPTOMS

- Patients will present with the classic symptoms of asthma:
  - Cough
  - Wheeze
  - Chest tightness
  - Shortness of breath.
- The patient may or may not link these symptoms to work, so it is important that the diagnosis is considered in all causes of new or worsening adult asthma.
- **Important points for history:**
  - A careful occupational history should be obtained including work duties, possible irritants, level of exposure, use of protective devices and any respiratory problems in colleagues.
  - Patients should be asked if their symptoms improve when they are not at work or on holiday.
  - Atopy is associated with occupational asthma.
  - Work-related rhinitis or conjunctivitis may be early signs of occupational asthma.
  - It is important to assess the level of exposure to potential allergens as this is a determinant of occupational asthma (See Table 15.1).
  - You should be aware that the latency period between exposure and developing symptoms can be up to several years in some cases.
- **Important point for examination:**
  - Expected examination findings will resemble those of asthma (see Chapter 3: Asthma).

5. INVESTIGATIONS

- Presence of asthma should be confirmed (see Chapter 3: Asthma).
- **Peak expiratory flow rate (PEFR):** The patient should keep a PEF diary taking recordings 4 times a day and noting when they are and are not at work.

Respiratory Medicine

Table 15.1 **Occupational exposures in asthma.**

EMPLOYMENT	AGENTS
Baking	Flour
Spray painting	Isocyanates
Laboratory animal work	Animal proteins
Healthcare	Latex Detergent enzymes Psyllium Glutaraldehyde (disinfectant) Methacrylates (joint replacement)
Food processing	Flour Seafood
Metalwork	Platinum, chromium, cobalt, nickel Soldering flux
Chemical processing	Phthalic anhydride (plastic production) Trimetallic anhydride (epoxy resin)
Woodwork	Red cedar Other wood dusts
Hairdressers and manicurists	Persulphates (hair bleach) Acrylates (artificial nails)

- Work-related asthma is suggested when there is a fall or increased variability of readings when at work, and improvement on days away from work.
- It is recommended that this should consist of a 2-week period at work and a 2-week period out of work.
- Serial PEF measurements can be statistically analysed to yield a numerical index value that predicts occupational asthma (see MICRO-Print, below).
- **Specific IgE levels and skin prick testing:** These tests can be used to test for sensitisation to suspected allergens.
    - This may be less useful in patients potentially sensitised to low-molecular-weight agents; these patients should be assessed via a specialist centre.
- **Specific inhalation challenge testing:** This is the gold standard test.
    - It is only available at certain centres, and a diagnosis can usually be made without this test.

> **MICRO-print**
> - Oasys is a free computer program available at www.occupational asthma.com.
> - It plots and interprets serial PEF measurements to give a computer-generated score between 1 and 4.
> - Scores >2.5 have a 75% sensitivity and 94% specificity for occupational asthma.

6. MANAGEMENT

- **Eliminate exposure to the antigen:** This is ideally undertaken through the removal of the agent from the workplace.
  - If this is not possible, the patient should be removed from the area of exposure.
  - Both of these measures may cause significant difficulties to the patient, and most patients are unable to resign from their jobs.
- **Minimise exposure to the antigen:** If elimination of exposure is not achievable.
  - This can be done by the use of respiratory protection equipment, ventilation in the workplace and monitoring the levels of the agent.
- **Pharmacological management:** This follows the asthma guidelines (see Chapter 3: Asthma).

7. PROGNOSIS

- Prognosis is related to the length of time and level of exposure to the allergen.
- The prognosis is improved in patients who have eliminated exposure to the allergen, who have good lung function at the time of diagnosis and a short history of symptoms prior to presentation.
- Symptoms are expected to substantially improve over the first year from removal of the causative agent.
- Two-thirds of patients never achieve symptomatic recovery, and three-quarters demonstrate ongoing non-specific bronchial hyper-responsiveness.
- There are profound economic implications for many patients with occupational asthma:
  - One-third of patients are unemployed up to six years after diagnosis.
  - Occupational asthma is covered by the industrial injuries disablement benefit.
  - The patient may make a civil claim against their employer if they failed to take action to protect them from harm.

Respiratory Medicine

15.2 ASBESTOSIS

1. DEFINITION

- Asbestosis is a pneumoconiosis (interstitial lung disease due to inorganic dust inhalation) caused by exposure to asbestos.
- Asbestos is a naturally occurring fibre composed of hydrated magnesium silicate.
- It was used extensively as a construction and insulation material before its health effects were understood.
- There may be a long latent period between the time of exposure and the onset of the disease.

2. EPIDEMIOLOGY

- In 2012, there were 216 deaths where asbestosis was recorded as the cause of death.
  - There were 464 deaths where asbestos is likely to have contributed.
- **High risk occupations:** Construction workers, joiners, plumbers, shipyard workers, railway workers, asbestos miners.
- Although non-occupational exposure to asbestos can occur, e.g. washing clothes of someone that works with asbestos, the cumulative exposure is usually insufficient to cause significant parenchymal asbestosis.

> **MICRO-references**
> Further epidemiological data is available from the Health and Safety Executive website: www.hse.gov.uk/statistics/causdis/asbestos-related-disease.pdf

3. AETIOLOGY

- Inhaled asbestos fibres are deposited at the bronchioles and alveolar ducts.
- Most fibres will be removed via the mucociliary escalator.
- Some fibres will be ingested by alveolar macrophages and type I cells.
- Lung damage may be due to directly toxic effects of the fibres on pulmonary cells or due to the release of mediators from inflammatory cells and formation of oxygen and nitrogen free radicals.

Respiratory Medicine

> **MICRO-print**
> **Asbestos fibres:**
> - Chrysolite (white) asbestos: the softest asbestos fibre.
>   - Fibres can be up to 2 cm long, but are typically only a few microns thick.
>   - It is the least fibrogenic asbestos.
> - Crocidolite (blue) asbestos: This asbestos fibre is most associated with lung disease.
>   - It is up to 50 mm in length and 1–2 μm wide and is particularly resistant to enzymatic destruction.
> - Amosite (brown) asbestos.
>   - Has intermediate fibrogenic properties.

4. CLINICAL FEATURES

- Asbestosis may be asymptomatic for $20-30$ years from the initial exposure.
- The more intense the exposure, the shorter the latent period.
- **Symptoms:**
  - Breathlessness.
  - Reduced exercise tolerance.
  - Cough and wheeze are not typical of asbestosis but may occur with co-existent smoking.
- **Signs:**
  - Fine end-inspiratory crackles on auscultation.
  - Finger clubbing.
  - Signs of cor pulmonale (late stage).

5. INVESTIGATIONS

- **Pulmonary function tests:**
  - Restrictive pattern of lung function.
  - Reduced lung volumes.
  - Reduced Tlco.
- **CXR:**
  - Bilateral interstitial changes in the lower zones in a reticular or multi-nodular pattern.
  - Presence of pleural plaques may suggest asbestosis rather than other fibrotic lung disease.
  - **Shaggy heart sign:** blurring of diaphragm and heart border.
  - Upper lobe involvement in advanced stages.
- **HRCT:** More sensitive in detecting asbestosis compared with plain radiographs.
  - Features similar to UIP (see chapter 12.1: Idiopathic pulmonary fibrosis).

Respiratory Medicine

- Mainly lower zone and subpleural changes initially.
- Honeycomb parenchymal changes.
- Traction bronchiectasis.

6. MANAGEMENT

- Prevention of further exposure to asbestos should be advised.
- Treat any co-existing COPD or cor pulmonale.
- Offer smoking cessation.
- Oxygen therapy for hypoxaemia.
- Pneumococcal and influenza vaccination.
- Treatment of respiratory infections.
- Some patients may be entitled to compensation and should seek guidance from the Department of Work and Pensions (see MICRO-Print, below).
- **Nintedanib:** In 2022 nintedanib was recommended for use in any progressive lung fibrosis. Evidence specifically for this condition is limited but it may reduce the rate of decline in FVC.

7. PROGNOSIS

- **Asbestosis may progress to respiratory failure. Risk factors for this include:**
  - Long duration of asbestos exposure.
  - Crocidolite exposure.
  - Severe symptoms.
  - Cigarette smoking.
  - Co-existent diffuse pleural thickening.
  - Honeycombing on HRCT.

MICRO-print

Compensation schemes for work-related lung diseases:

- Industrial injuries disablement benefit:
  - A weekly benefit paid to individuals with asbestosis/pneumoconiosis whose exposure occurred while in employment.
  - Individuals who were self-employed when the exposure occurred are not entitled to it.
- Civil claim for compensation through the courts.
  - A claim for a lump compensation sum under the Pneumoconiosis etc. (Workers' Compensation) Act 1979.
  - Paid to individuals with asbestosis/pneumoconiosis who are unable to claim compensation through the courts because the employer is no longer trading.
  - If the individual exposed has died from the condition, their dependents can claim compensation under this act.

15.3 ASBESTOS-RELATED PLEURAL DISEASES

1. DEFINITION

- Asbestos exposure can cause a number of diseases of the pleura including pleural plaques, pleural thickening, benign asbestos-related pleural effusions (BAPE), and malignant mesothelioma (see Chapter 5: Lung Malignancy).

2. EPIDEMIOLOGY

- Pleural plaques develop in ~ 50% of people exposed to asbestos.
- In 2013, there were 430 new cases of pleural thickening assessed for Industrial Injuries Disablement Benefit.

3. PATHOPHYSIOLOGY

- Pleural plaques and diffuse pleural thickening occur when inhaled asbestos fibres become embedded in the pleural space.
- Injury due to the asbestos fibres activates fibroblasts and mesothelial cells causing fibrosis, calcification, scarring and thickening.
- Pleural plaques are the result of localised fibrosis and are typically asymptomatic.
- Diffuse pleural thickening is more widespread and as a consequence can result in restriction in lung expansion.
- Pleural plaques typically affect the parietal pleura adjacent to the ribs. They are most commonly found in the sixth to ninth ribs and along the diaphragm.

4. CLINICAL FEATURES

- **Pleural plaques:**
    - Typically asymptomatic but may cause chest pain in a small minority of patients.
    - Plaques themselves do not transform into malignant lesions but their presence should raise the possibility of mesothelioma.
- **Diffuse pleural thickening:**
    - May result in breathlessness.
    - Chest pain has been reported in some patients.
- **Benign asbestos-related pleural effusions (BAPE):**
    - Large effusions may cause breathlessness, requiring drainage.

5. INVESTIGATIONS

- **CXR:**
    - **Pleural plaques:**
        - Bilateral, irregular, well-defined opacities.
        - There may be evidence of associated pleural thickening.

- **Diffuse pleural thickening:**
  - A continuous pleural density affecting 25% of the chest wall.
  - Blunting of the costophrenic angles.
- **HRCT:**
  - Useful to differentiate pleural plaques from solid tumours.
  - **Diffuse pleural thickening:** A continuous sheet of pleural thickening >5 cm wide, >8 cm long and >3 mm thick.
- **Lung function tests:**
  - May show a restrictive defect in diffuse pleural thickening with reduced static lung volumes and Tlco.
- **Biopsy** of pleural plaques may be required to exclude mesothelioma.

6. MANAGEMENT

- Pleural plaques do not require routine CT scan assessment or follow-up.
- Smoking cessation should be offered.
- BAPE should be a diagnosis of exclusion and may require thoracoscopy to drain fluid and allow adequate pleural biopsies to exclude potential mesothelioma.
- Pleural thickening may require serial follow-up with spirometry and CXR/CT follow-up to look for progression.
- There may be a very small role for surgery in diffuse pleural thickening.

15.4 COAL WORKERS PNEUMOCONIOSIS

1. DEFINITION

- Coal workers pneumoconiosis (CWP) is a fibrotic lung disease caused by inhalation of coal dust. It is now relatively uncommon due to changes in working practices.
- It is divided into:
  - **Simple coal workers pneumoconiosis:** a largely asymptomatic condition characterised by nodules on chest X-ray.
  - **Progressive massive fibrosis (PMF):** a nodular, fibrotic disorder which causes symptoms and may progress to lung failure.

2. EPIDEMIOLOGY

- In 2013, 275 new cases of CWP were assessed for Industrial Injuries and Disablement Benefit.
- There were 140 deaths from CWP in 2012.

3 AETIOLOGY

- The carbon from inhaled coal dust is ingested by macrophages.
- Under normal circumstances, these phagocytosed coal dust particles are transported out of the lungs via the mucociliary escalator.

- Continued inhalation of coal dust may overwhelm this defence mechanism, resulting in accumulation of coal dust-laden macrophages in the alveoli.
- This triggers an immune response in the lungs.
- Fibroblasts lay down reticulin, resulting in fibrosis.
- This process is accelerated by macrophage lysis, e.g. if the coal has a high silica content (see section 15.5, Silicosis).

4. CLINICAL FEATURES

- **Symptoms:**
  - Simple coal workers pneumoconiosis:
    - Often asymptomatic in the early stages.
    - Can accelerate/increase the risk of COPD.
  - Progressive massive fibrosis:
    - Shortness of breath on exertion.
    - Cough.
    - Black sputum.
  - **Important points in the history:**
    - Age at first exposure.
    - Duration of exposure.
    - Type of coal mined and silica content.
    - Any smoking history?

MICRO-print

Caplan Syndrome

- Coal workers pneumoconiosis in association with rheumatoid arthritis is called Caplan syndrome.
- Radiological findings are bilateral, peripheral nodules 5 mm to 5 cm in size.
- Caplan syndrome may progress more rapidly than simple pneumoconiosis.
- Lesions may cavitate or calcify.

---

5. INVESTIGATIONS

- **Chest X-ray:**
  - Small rounded nodular opacities, typically in the upper lobes.
  - **PMF:** Confluence of these nodules and development of large opacities.
- **Pulmonary function tests:** These show a mixed obstructive/restrictive pattern in PMF.
- **CT:**
  - Lung nodules mainly perilymphatic and in the upper zones.
  - Nodules can be calcified.

Respiratory Medicine

> **MICRO-print**
>
> The International Labour Organization (ILO) International Classification of Radiographs of Pneumoconioses is used throughout the world for health surveillance, research and statistical analysis (www.ilo.org/safe-work/info/WCMS_108548/lang-en/index.htm).
>
> Radiological classification of CWP:
>
> - Lung zones are divided into upper, middle and lower zones.
> - Parenchymal opacities on the CXR are classified as:
>   - P: <1.5 mm in diameter
>   - Q: 1.5–3 mm in diameter
>   - R: >3 to 10 mm in diameter.
> - Nodules >1 cm define complicated CWP or PMF:
>   - A: Any opacity 1–5 cm in diameter.
>   - B: Opacity >5 cm, occupying <1/3 of the lung.
>   - C: Opacity exceeding >1/3 total area of the lung.

6. MANAGEMENT

- Management of CWP and PMF is largely symptomatic.
- Remove from dust exposure.
- Smoking cessation.
- Oxygen therapy.
- As with asbestosis, some patients may be entitled to compensation (see MICRO-Print Box: "Compensation schemes for work-related lung diseases" above).

15.5 SILICOSIS

1. DEFINITION

- A disease caused by the inhalation of silica (silicon dioxide) – an inorganic mineral found in stone and sand.

2. EPIDEMIOLOGY

- Silicosis is relatively uncommon.
    - In 2013, there were 45 new cases of silicosis assessed for Industrial Injuries and Disablement Benefit.
    - In 2012, there were 11 deaths due to silicosis.
- Occupations at risk of exposure: stone masons, sand-blasters, pottery/ceramic workers, some foundry workers and glass workers.

3. PATHOPHYSIOLOGY

- Inhaled silica is ingested by macrophages. However, it is toxic to macrophages.
- This results in macrophage death and the release of proteolytic enzymes and undigested silica.
- Proteolytic enzymes cause local tissue destruction and fibrosis.
- The released silica particles are then re-ingested by further macrophages, thus repeating the cycle.

4. CLINICAL FEATURES

- Shortness of breath
- Cough
- Fever
- Cyanosis in respiratory failure.

5. INVESTIGATIONS

- **Chest X-Ray**
  - **Similar appearance to CWP:** Small rounded opacities in the upper lobes.
  - Confluence of these opacities can result in the formation of opacities >1 cm in size.
  - Hilar lymph node enlargement may be evident.
  - **Eggshell calcification:** thin streaks of calcification around hilar lymph nodes.
- **HRCT:**
  - More sensitive than CXR.
  - This shows bilateral, symmetric, centrilobular and perilymphatic nodules, which may calcify.
  - Emphysematous changes may be evident in complicated silicosis.

6. MANAGEMENT

Management of silicosis is symptomatic, as with CWP.

Some patients may be entitled to compensation (see MICRO-Print Box: "Compensation schemes for work-related lung diseases" above).

There is a strongly elevated risk of tuberculosis with radiological silicosis which should be borne in mind especially if symptoms change or worsen.

Respiratory Medicine

MICRO-case

You are a respiratory physician working in a busy outpatient clinic, when you see a 70-year-old man, Mr. Turner, who has been suffering with shortness of breath on exertion for the past few months. He has no associated cough or wheeze. Examination reveals fine bibasal lung crackles but no other significant positive findings.

His GP has arranged a chest X-ray and pulmonary function test prior to the appointment. The chest X-ray shows bilateral lower zone interstitial changes and pleural plaques, in addition to areas of pleural thickening. Pulmonary function tests arranged pre-clinic demonstrate reduced FEV_1 and FVC, reduced static lung volumes and reduced Tlco.

On review of his history, you discover that he had heavy exposure to asbestos whilst working as a plumber.

You suspect asbestosis and arrange an outpatient CT scan.

You advise him that there is no specific treatment for his condition but encourage him to stop smoking and refer him to the smoking cessation and pulmonary rehabilitation services. Post clinic CT scan highlights pleural plaques and lung fibrosis consistent with asbestosis.

Mr. Turner is entitled to compensation under the Pneumoconiosis etc. (Workers' Compensation) Act 1979 as his illness was caused by exposure to asbestos during his employment and the company has ceased trading.

Key Points

- The presence of pleural changes in addition to interstitial disease is suggestive of asbestosis.
- Detailed history taking is vital to identify occupational exposure.
- Management of asbestosis (and other pneumoconioses) is supportive.
- Patients (and in some cases their relatives) can claim industrial compensation via a number of routes.

16 Respiratory Emergencies

16.1 RESPIRATORY FAILURE

1. AETIOLOGY

- **Type 1 respiratory failure:** Hypoxia ($P_aO_2 < 8kPa$ when breathing room air) with normal or low $PaCO_2$.
  - V/Q mismatch:
    - Pneumonia
    - Pulmonary oedema
    - PE
    - Asthma
    - COPD.
  - Diffusion defect
    - Interstitial lung disease
    - Emphysema.
  - Right-to-left shunt (does not improve with supplemental oxygen)
    - Arteriovenous malformation
    - Severe pneumonia
    - Lung collapse.
- **Type 2 respiratory failure:** Hypoxia $(P_aO_2 < 8kPa)$ with hypercapnia $(PaCO_2 > 6.0kPa)$.
  - Respiratory pump failure (hypoventilation).
    - Reduced respiratory drive due to CNS disease or sedative drugs.
    - Neuromuscular disease (MND, Guillain-Barré, myasthenia gravis, spinal cord injury).
    - Chest wall and pleural disorders (flail chest, kyphoscoliosis, obesity, severe hyperinflation).
  - Increased dead space (areas of the lung that are not anatomically or physiologically able to exchange gas) ventilation is the main mechanism in COPD and is exacerbated by tachypnoea.

DOI: 10.1201/9781315113937-17

2. INVESTIGATIONS

- **Pulse oximetry:**
  - Reliable for measuring oxygen saturations but may overestimate oxygen levels in patients with darker skin tones.
- **Blood gas analysis:**
  - This gives more accurate measurement of oxygenation but also provides information on $pCO2$, acid-base status and other results.
  - Gold standard is an arterial blood gas but this is more invasive and often painful for patients.
  - Venous blood gases are usually reliable if the venous $O2$ saturation is $> 75\%$.
  - Capillary blood gases (taken by "arterialising" blood from the earlobe using a rubefacient) is often used if multiple measurements needed in a patient without an arterial line.

3. IMMEDIATE MANAGEMENT

- **Always begin with an ABCDE (airway, breathing, circulation, disability and exposure) approach in the unwell patient.**
- **Consider whether admission to a critical care setting is appropriate:** often necessary in acute respiratory failure.
- **Type 1 failure:**
  - Aim for oxygen saturations of 94–98%.
  - Deliver oxygen at 2–4 L/min by nasal cannula; or FiO_2 $24 - 60\%$ via Venturi mask.
  - If $SpO_2 < 85\%$ use oxygen at 15 L/min via a non-rebreathable mask.
  - Take a blood gas at the earliest opportunity:
    - **If PaO_2 and $PaCO_2$ are above or within the normal range:** consider reducing flow rate/concentration.
    - **If PaO_2 remains <8kPa despite 60% O_2 :** Consider critical care support: CPAP (continuous positive airway pressure) or intubation.
  - Treat underlying cause.
- **Type 2 failure:**
  - **Critical to consider whether this is acute or chronic.**
    - Chronic type 2 respiratory failure is suggested by a normal pH with a raised bicarbonate and positive base excess – this is not an emergency.
    - Acute type 2 respiratory failure is suggested by a low pH or a signifi cant rise in $pCO2$ above a previous baseline.
  - Aim for baseline oxygen saturations of $88 - 92\%$.

- Controlled oxygen therapy, beginning at $24\% \ O_2$, via Venturi mask.
- **Recheck ABG after 20 mins:**
  - If pH and $PaCO_2$ are within normal limits and $pO_2 > 8kPa$, aim for target saturations of $94 - 98\%$. Repeat ABG analysis in $30 - 60$ minutes.
  - If previous history of severe type 2 respiratory failure then target saturations of $88 - 92\%$. may be more appropriate.
    - Aim for $88 - 92\%$. saturations if pH is within normal limits but CO_2 is raised.
  - If controlled oxygen therapy and active management of the underlying condition fails, consider NIV or invasive ventilation.
- The exception to this approach is in a deteriorating patient who develops a rising $pCO2$ during treatment for type 1 respiratory failure – for example in acute severe asthma.
  - This can be an indication of respiratory muscle fatigue and should prompt immediate consideration of assisted ventilation.
  - Reducing the inspired oxygen concentration in this scenario is likely to hasten deterioration.

16.2 ACUTE ASTHMA

1. CLINICAL FEATURES

- **In life-threatening asthma:**
  - PEFR (peak expiratory flow rate) <33% predicted/best.
  - $SaO_2 < 92\%$.
  - $Pa \ O_2 < 8kPa$.
  - Normal CO_2.
  - Silent chest.
  - Cyanosis.
  - Poor respiratory effort.
  - Bradycardia/arrhythmia/hypotension.
  - Exhaustion.
  - Confusion.
  - Coma.

2. IMMEDIATE MANAGEMENT

- For moderate/severe acute asthma exacerbations and continuing management, see Chapter 3: Asthma.
- Immediate management of life threatening asthma is summarised as a flowchart in Figure 16.1.

Respiratory Medicine

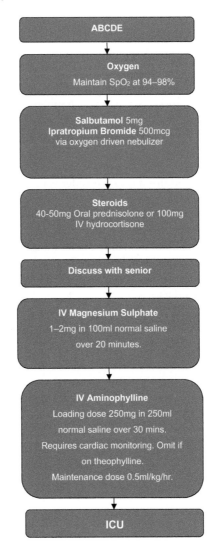

Figure 16.1 Management of life-threatening status asthmaticus.

16.3 COPD EXACERBATION

1. AETIOLOGY

- **Exacerbations in COPD may be:**
  - Infective
  - Non-infective.

2. CLINICAL FEATURES

- **Increased symptoms of COPD**
  - Cough
  - Worsening in sputum characteristics
  - Breathlessness
  - Wheeze
  - Decreased exercise capacity.

3. IMMEDIATE MANAGEMENT

- Immediate management of severe COPD exacerbation is summarised as a flowchart in Figure 16.2.

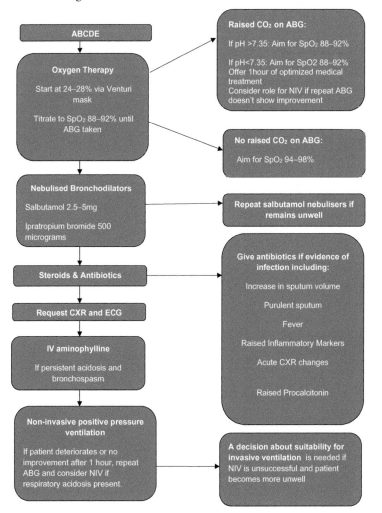

Figure 16.2 Management of severe COPD exacerbation.

16.4 ANAPHYLAXIS

1. AETIOLOGY

- Type 1 IgE-mediated hypersensitivity reaction.
- **Common precipitants:**
  - Drugs
  - Eggs
  - Shellfish
  - Peanuts and other nuts
  - Stings/insect bites.

2. CLINICAL FEATURES

MICRO-facts

Anaphylaxis is likely in the presence of the following features:

1. Sudden onset and rapidly progressing clinical features.
2. Airway/breathing/circulation compromise.
3. Skin and/or mucosal changes.
4. +/− exposure to a known trigger.

- **Skin/mucosal changes:** Itching, erythema, oedema, urticaria.
- **Airway problems:** Wheeze, laryngeal obstruction, stridor.
- **Breathing problems:** SOB, wheeze, confusion, cyanosis, fatigue, respiratory arrest.
- **Circulatory problems (shock):** Hypotension, tachycardia, sweating, pallor, dizziness, cardiac arrest.
- **GI symptoms:** May be present e.g. diarrhoea and vomiting.

3. IMMEDIATE MANAGEMENT

- See Figure 16.3.

Respiratory Medicine

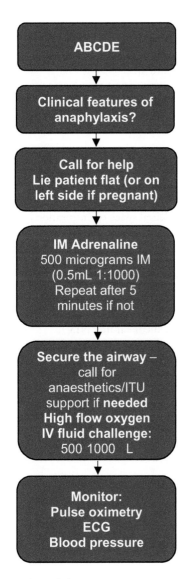

Figure 16.3 Management of anaphylaxis.

> **MICRO-references**
> Flowcharts adapted from the Resuscitation Council UK Anaphylaxis guidelines 2021, available at:
> www.resus.org.uk/library/additional-guidance/guidance-anaphylaxis/emergency-treatment

16.5 TENSION PNEUMOTHORAX

1. AETIOLOGY

- Air is drawn into the pleural space on inspiration but has no means of escape on expiration.
  - The increase in volume pushes the mediastinum into the contralateral hemithorax.
  - Compression of the great veins occurs.
  - Death by cardiorespiratory arrest will occur if not decompressed.
- **Situations in which tension pneumothorax may arise:**
  - In ventilated patients (including NIV).
  - Following trauma.
  - With pre-existing respiratory disease:
    - Asthma
    - COPD.
  - During cardiopulmonary resuscitation.
  - Due to blocked, clamped or displaced chest drains.

2. CLINICAL FEATURES

- Tachycardia.
- Reduced chest expansion.
- Hyper-resonant percussion note.
- Reduced breath sounds.
- Deviation of the trachea towards contralateral lung.
- Displacement of the apex beat.
- Hypotension and collapse.

3. IMMEDIATE MANAGEMENT

- If tension pneumothorax is suspected and patient is critically ill, action may be required in absence of CXR confirmation.
- If patient is unwell (significant respiratory distress +/– haemodynamic compromise), consider urgent needle decompression (see Figure 16.4):

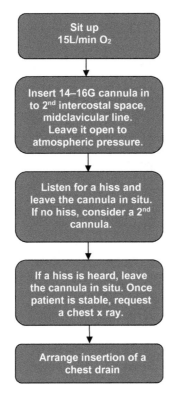

Figure 16.4 Management of tension pneumothorax.

16.6 MASSIVE PULMONARY EMBOLUS (PE)

1. AETIOLOGY

- In massive PE, a significant thrombus burden causes right heart strain and impaired filling of left ventricle, leading to haemodynamic compromise.
- Defined by PE with hypotension (<90 mmHg), postural hypotension or syncope. Submassive PE occurs without hypotension but with evidence of right heart strain on CT-PA or echocardiography, and/or serum markers of myocardial injury.

2. CLINICAL FEATURES

- Clinical features:
  - Clinical history of PE (see Chapter 7) with symptoms of syncope, or presenting with shock.
  - Tachypnoea.

- Hypoxia.
- Tachycardia.
- Pale.
- Clammy.
- Poor capillary refill.
- Hypotension, including postural drop >20 mmHg SBP.
- Gallop rhythm.
- Increased JVP.
- Laboratory features:
  - Elevated serum troponin
  - Raised serum lactate
- CTPA radiological features:
  - Extensive thrombus burden within main lobar branches.
  - Straightening of interventricular septum.
  - Enlarged right ventricle.
- Consider risk factors (see Chapter 7: Pulmonary Embolism).

3. IMMEDIATE MANAGEMENT

- The major risk of thrombolysis is bleeding, including intracranial bleeds.

MICRO-facts

Contraindications to systemic thrombolysis
- Absolute:
  - Ischaemic stroke in last 6 months.
  - Haemorrhagic stroke at any time.
  - GI bleeding in last month.
  - Known bleeding.
  - CNS neoplasm.
- Relative:
  - TIA in last 6 months.
  - Malignancy.
  - Oral anticoagulation.
  - Pregnancy or within 1 week post-partum.
  - Non-compressible punctures.
  - Traumatic resuscitation.
  - Advanced liver disease.
  - Infective endocarditis.
  - Active peptic ulcer.

● Immediate management of massive PE is summarised as a flowchart in Figure 16.5.

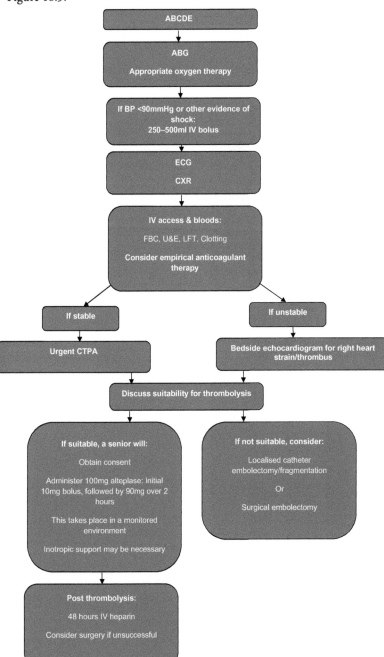

Figure 16.5 Management of massive PE.

16.7 MASSIVE HAEMOPTYSIS

1. DEFINITION

- Haemoptysis is the coughing of blood originating in the respiratory tract below the larynx.
- A number of thresholds for "massive" haemoptysis have been proposed.
- These range from 100 *to* $600mL$ lost in 24 hours.
- The risk of death is from respiratory compromise, rather than hypovolaemia or shock.

2. AETIOLOGY

- Typically the bleed arises from the bronchial circulation, which is a higher pressure system than the pulmonary circulation.
- Bleeds from the pulmonary circulation can arise from arteriovenous (AV) malformations.
- **Specific causes:**
  - Tuberculosis (Rasmussen's aneurysm)
  - Bronchiectasis
  - Lung abscess
  - Aspergillosis
  - Cystic fibrosis
  - Neoplasia
  - Pulmonary embolism
  - Vasculitis
  - Trauma:
    - Pulmonary artery catheter
    - Penetrating external
    - Blunt external.
  - Arteriovenous malformation
  - Cardiac valve disease:
    - Mitral stenosis
    - Infective endocarditis.
  - Coagulopathy.

3. MANAGEMENT

- Massive haemoptysis is a medical emergency.
- **Immediate management:**
  - **Resuscitate according to "ABC" approach.**
    - Position the patient on the affected side if the bleeding point is known – this will allow a tamponade effect.
    - High-flow oxygen and suction.

- Secure the airway: may require intubation with a double lumen tube.
  ○ An anaesthetist with suitable expertise may able to attempt tamponade with a Foley catheter via the endotracheal tube.
- Transfuse based on haemodynamic parameters, not blood lost.
- Reverse any coagulopathy or thrombocytopenia, stop antiplatelet and anticoagulant drugs.
- Tranexamic acid is effective (can be given IV/PO or nebulised).
- **Localise the bleeding site.**
  - CXR followed by CT with contrast.
  - Bronchoscopy.
- **Angiography and embolisation:** embolisation of the bronchial artery.
  - Usually considered if initial management fails to control the bleeding, or if there is a high risk of rebleeding.
  - Used in AV malformations as a definitive treatment or before surgery can be performed.
  - Small risk of spinal cord infarction.
- **Bronchoscopic therapy:**
  - **Iced saline lavage:** causes vasospasm.
  - **Topical agents:** adrenaline, thrombin or fibrinogen-thrombin glue.
  - Endobronchial balloon catheter tamponade.
  - Laser photocoagulation.
- **Surgical management:**
  - Segmentectomy
  - Lobectomy
  - Pneumonectomy.
- **Radiotherapy:**
  - If malignancy is the underlying cause.

16.8 SUPERIOR VENA CAVA OBSTRUCTION (SVCO)

. AETIOLOGY

Superior vena cava obstruction (SVCO) occurs due to an intrinsic obstruction or extrinsic pressure on the SVC wall.
Can be supra- or infra-azygous.
- Infra-azygous is more severe.
Specific causes:
- **Primary bronchial carcinoma:** the most common cause (~75% of malignant SVC cases).
- **Lymphoma:** ~12% of malignant SVC cases.

Respiratory Medicine

- Thymoma.
- Germ cell tumours.
- Metastatic disease.
- Aortic aneurysm.
- **Mediastinal fibrosis:**
  - Infections
  - Radiotherapy.
- **SVC thrombosis:**
  - Central venous catheter.
  - Pacemaker or implantable cardiac defibrillator leads.

2. CLINICAL FEATURES

- Plethoric.
- Swollen face.
- Dilated chest collateral vessels.
- Arm swelling.
- ↑JVP – non-pulsatile.
- Dyspnoea.
- Papilloedema.
- **Pemberton's test:** lift arms above head for >1 min; a positive result is development of facial plethora or cyanosis.

3. INVESTIGATIONS

- **Chest X-ray:** widened mediastinum or mass in right hemithorax.
- **CT scan:** with contrast.
- **Doppler scan:** use to evaluate the severity of obstruction and effect of therapy.
- **Invasive contrast venography.**

4. MANAGEMENT

- Elevate the head.
- Give oxygen if hypoxic.
- High-dose dexamethasone (8 mg BD) is usually given with proton pump inhibitor (PPI) cover (although this is often of limited efficacy).
- Stenting the SVC is appropriate in SVCO if the patient is very symptomatic, although may be deferred if treatment of the underlying cause is expected to be successful.
- Consider low-molecular-weight heparin (LMWH) to prevent thrombosis.
- Aim to confirm diagnosis.
- **Treatment of the underlying disease.**
  - Radiotherapy for most malignancies.
  - Urgent chemotherapy if small cell lung cancer.
  - Lymphoma should respond to dexamethasone in the short term.
  - Anticoagulants for central venous thrombosis.

MICRO-case

You are the SHO on nights at a district general hospital when you are called to see a 75-year-old patient who has become acutely short of breath over the last few minutes. The staff nurse responsible for the patient explains that she became acutely short of breath after receiving a dose of amoxicillin for a presumed pneumonia. She has no documented history of penicillin allergy and has never been in hospital before. As this patient has acutely deteriorated, you use the ABCDE approach to examine her:

A: Patent, patient speaking in short sentences, no evidence of stridor.
B: Dyspnoeic, respiratory rate is 26, wheeze on auscultation.
C: BP – 110/65 (her normal BP is ~140/80). Heart rate – 112 bpm.
D: GCS 15/15. BMs normal.
E: Urticarial rash (wheals) around the cannula site.

You recognise a case of anaphylaxis and begin acute management, asking a nurse to call the medical emergencies team. While you wait for them to arrive, you administer high-flow oxygen, insert a large-bore cannula and administer 0.5 mL of 1:1000 adrenaline via the intramuscular route. The shortness of breath resolves over a few minutes. You pre-scribe 500 mL normal saline. When the medical emergency team arrive, the patient has stabilised and the medical registrar commends your management!

Key Points

- Always use the ABCDE approach when assessing the acutely unwell patient. You should also use this approach to document your findings in the notes.
- The clinical picture is more relevant in recognising anaphylaxis than a documented allergy or known trigger.
  - Suspect anaphylaxis if there is a rapid onset of airway, breathing or circulatory problems associated with skin or mucosal changes.
- Always interpret vital signs in the context of the patient's normal values.
  - In this case a systolic BP of 110 may have been falsely reassuring if the previous trend had not been noted.
- It is better to call the medical emergency team early in a potentially life-threatening situation! The aim is to prevent, as well as manage, cardiac arrest.

Respiratory Medicine

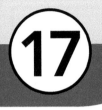

17 Smoking and the Lung

1. EPIDEMIOLOGY

- In the UK the number of people who smoke is decreasing, however a significant proportion of people still smoke.
  - In 2021, 13% of UK adults smoked which equates to an estimated 7 million UK adult cigarette smokers (see MICRO-References, below)
  - Two thirds of smokers start before the age of 18.
  - Smoking rates are higher in lower socio-economic groups.

MICRO-references
www.ons.gov.uk/peoplepopulationandcommunity/healthandsocialcare/
healthandlifeexpectancies/bulletins/adultsmokinghabitsin
greatbritain/2021

2. COST TO THE NHS

- Smoking costs the NHS in England an estimated £2.6 billion a year.
- In 2015/16, £145 million was spent on prescriptions to help stop smoking.
- In 2015/16, 520,000 hospital admissions were directly attributable to smoking.

MICRO-reference
www.gov.uk/government/publications/cost-of-smoking-to-the-nhs-in-england-2015/cost-of-smoking-to-the-nhs-in-england-2015

DOI: 10.1201/9781315113937-18

3. MORTALITY

- Smoking is the largest cause of preventable and premature death in the UK, and is greater than all the next 6 causes put together.
  - There are $100,000$ deaths a year in the UK due to smoking, and 6 million deaths a year globally.
  - Roughly 50% of smokers will die of smoking-related illness.
- After the age of 35, every year of smoking reduces life expectancy by 3 months.
- On average, smokers die 10 years earlier than non-smokers.

4. LUNG DISEASE ASSOCIATED WITH SMOKING

- Smoking causes 36% of all respiratory deaths; it is implicated in the following respiratory illnesses:
  - Lung cancer
    - 80% of lung cancer deaths are attributable to smoking.
  - COPD
    - Smoking accounts for 90% of COPD cases, and $30-40\%$ of smokers develop COPD.
    - Patients who continue to smoke have a greater rate of lung function decline and poorer outcomes.
  - Pneumonia
    - There is higher risk in both passive and active smokers.
  - TB
    - Smoking is a risk factor for developing TB. Furthermore, smokers with TB have a higher mortality rate.
  - Asthma.
    - Exacerbates asthma symptoms, causing higher rates of hospitalisation.
    - Reduces the effectiveness of inhaled corticosteroids.
    - Exposure to secondhand smoke is a trigger for the development of childhood asthma and leads to increased symptomatology.

5. EXTRA-PULMONARY DISEASE

- Smoking is implicated in cancers other than lung including oral, bladder, breast, renal, gastric, liver and cervical cancers.
- The extra-pulmonary health effects of smoking are listed in Table 17.1.

Respiratory Medicine

Table 17.1 **Extra-pulmonary health effects of smoking.**

EXTRA-PULMONARY ORGAN SYSTEMS EFFECTED BY SMOKING	DISEASES DIRECTLY ATTRIBUTABLE TO OR STRONGLY ASSOCIATED WITH SMOKING
Cardiovascular disease	• Chronic heart disease. • Myocardial infarction. • Angina pectoralis. • Peripheral vascular disease. • 17% of all cardiovascular disease deaths are attributable to smoking. • Increased risk of abdominal aortic aneurysm and rupture.
Cerebrovascular disease	• 10% of deaths from stroke are attributable to smoking. • Increased risk of intracranial aneurysm.
Gastrointestinal disease	• Gastric cancer. • Duodenal and gastric ulcers. • Colonic polyps. • Crohn's disease.
Oropharyngeal disease	• Poor dentition. • Head and neck cancers.
Eye disease	• Cataracts. • Macular degeneration. • Optic neuropathy.
Reproductive organs	• Impaired female fertility. • Earlier onset of menopause. • Increased rates of cervical and breast cancer. • Reduced sperm count and increased rate of impotence. • Neonatal complications: • Premature birth. • Low birth weight. • Preterm related death. • Sudden infant death syndrome.

6. BRIEF INTERVENTION

- Two-thirds of smokers want to stop smoking.
- Brief interventions allow health care professionals to give opportunistic advice to smokers in a 5–10 minute consultation.

Respiratory Medicine

- Brief interventions are evidence based and cost-effective.
- Brief intervention alone leads to 5% of smokers stopping smoking for 6 months.
- Multiple interventions have a "dripping tap" effect of encouraging patients to quit over a long period of time
- The number needed to treat for brief intervention to prevent one premature death is 80, rising to 16 − 40 when behavioural support is added. This compares extremely favourably with commonly prescribed preventative medications for other major health problems.
- It should consist of 5 elements as presented in Figure 17.1:

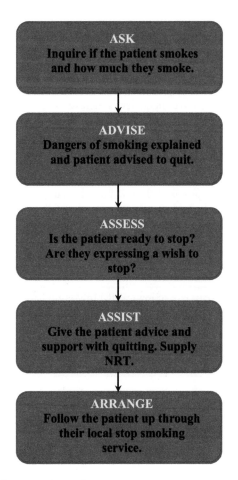

ASK
Inquire if the patient smokes and how much they smoke.

ADVISE
Dangers of smoking explained and patient advised to quit.

ASSESS
Is the patient ready to stop? Are they expressing a wish to stop?

ASSIST
Give the patient advice and support with quitting. Supply NRT.

ARRANGE
Follow the patient up through their local stop smoking service.

Figure 17.1 Smoking cessation pathway.

- If the patient does not want to, or is not ready to quit, advise them where they can get help if they change their mind in the future.
- The health benefits of smoking cessation are listed in Table 17.2.

Table 17.2 **Benefits of stopping smoking.**

TIME AFTER STOPPING SMOKING	HEALTH BENEFITS
20 minutes	• Blood pressure and heart rate return to normal.
8 hours	• Nicotine levels reduced by 90%. • Carbon monoxide levels reduce by 75%.
48 hours	• Carbon monoxide eliminated from body. • Lungs start to clear mucus and debris. • Nicotine eliminated from the body. • Ability to taste and smell improved.
72 hours	• Patients report breathing is easier • Subjective energy levels increase.
2–12 weeks	• Reduced rate of respiratory infections. • Symptoms of coughing and shortness of breath improve. • Physical appearance improves. • Reduced severity of asthma attacks.
3–9 months	• Symptoms of chronic bronchitis improve. • Risk of duodenal or gastric ulcer falls. • Lung function improvement for patients with mild/moderate COPD.
1 year	• An ex smoker previously smoking 20/day will have saved in excess of £3000.
5 years	• Excess risk of myocardial infarction halves. • Decline in lung function equals that of a never-smoker.
10 years	• Risk of lung cancer falls to 50% of the risk of a smoker. • Risk of myocardial infarction falls to that of a never-smoker.

7. SMOKING CESSATION COUNSELLING

- Support from stop smoking services can be delivered by:
  - Group sessions.
  - Drop-in sessions.
  - Telephone consultations.
  - Individual appointments with a specialist stop smoking practitioner.
- The quit rate at 1 year after smoking cessation intervention is 15%, compared to 4% of people who stop unaided.

> **MICRO-print**
>
> Quitting smoking is a difficult process: 85% of smokers who try to quit relapse within a week. Smokers go through 7 stages or psychological processes of quitting.
>
> 1. Pre-contemplation: Smoking is not considered a problem to the patient.
> 2. Contemplation: The patient starts to consider quitting.
> 3. Preparation: The patient wants to quit and starts planning a quit date.
> 4. Action: The patient stops smoking.
> 5. Maintenance: The patient continues to avoid smoking.
> 6. Termination: The patient no longer craves tobacco.
> 7. Relapse: Most commonly smokers progress to this stage; it usually takes at least 4 attempts to quit.

3. NICOTINE REPLACEMENT THERAPY (NRT)

- A combination of NRT with counselling increases quit rates to 25%.
  - NRT is designed to minimise the effects of nicotine withdrawal.
  - It can be prescribed, and most are available as over-the-counter medications; there are multiple preparations available.
  - Most preparations are taken for 8–12 weeks.
- Long-acting preparations such as patches can be used in combination with rapid-acting preparations:
  - Patches
  - Chewing gum
  - Sublingual tablets
  - Lozenges
  - Inhalator
  - Nasal spray.

4. OTHER SUPPORTIVE PHARMACOTHERAPY

- Bupropion (Zyban):
  - Counteracts nicotine withdrawal symptoms by inhibiting dopamine, serotonin and noradrenaline uptake, thus increasing the levels in the brain.
  - It has shown to lead to a 30% quit rate at 12 months when combined with counselling.
- Varenicline (Champix):
  - Binds to and has a partial agonist effect to the a4b2-nicotine acetylcholine receptors, thus lessening the symptoms of withdrawal and reducing the rewarding effects of smoking.
  - 22% quit rate at 12 months.

Respiratory Medicine

- Both bupropion and varenicline are prescription-only medicines and should only be prescribed in patients with a firm quit date and with counselling arranged for ongoing follow-up.
- These drugs can cause behavioural disturbance, especially with regards to suicidal ideation, and should therefore be used with extreme caution in adolescents.

MICRO-facts

Risk vs Reward: Contraindications of Smoking Cessation Medication
Varenicline:

- Do not use in patients with a history of depression or serious neuro-psychiatric conditions; safety has not been established in this patient group.
    - Increases risk of depression, suicidal ideation and completed suicide.
    - Any patient reporting neuro-psychiatric symptoms should have the drug stopped permanently.
- Seizures due to the drug reported. Use with caution in patients with a history of seizure or seizure disorders.
- Increased risk cardiovascular events and cardiovascular-related death. Use with caution if history is suggestive of arteriopathy.

Bupropion:

- Lowers the seizure threshold, is contraindicated in patients at risk of developing seizures. Previous seizures are an absolute contraindication.
- Contraindicated in patients with history of anorexia nervosa or bulimia. Medication can cause significant weight loss.

MICRO-print

- Electronic nicotine delivery system or e-cigarettes are increasingly being used by smokers to quit.
- They are widely used and have been shown to aid quitting of tobacco compared to placebo.
- Their use has generated controversy:
    - The long-term impact on health is uncertain.
    - There is concern that they could be used to attract a new generation into smoking and nicotine addiction.
- However, the majority consensus is that these products carry far less risk than tobacco.

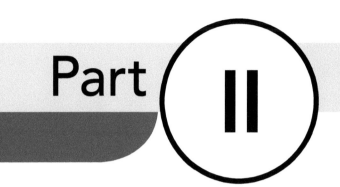

Part **II**

Questions and Answers

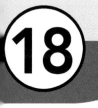

Questions and Answers

Questions

CHAPTER 1: CLINICAL ASSESSMENT

EMQ: Lung function test

1. Asbestosis
2. Asthma
3. Bronchiectasis
4. Coal workers pneumoconiosis
5. COPD

6. Drug-induced pulmonary fibrosis
7. Farmer's lung
8. Idiopathic pulmonary fibrosis
9. Normal lung function
10. Pigeon fanciers lung

Question 1

You are the junior doctor on the respiratory ward and have been asked to review the spirometry results of a 45-year-old woman. She has a history of rheumatoid arthritis and takes a number of anti-rheumatic drugs. The results show:

	RESULTS
FEV$_1$ (% predicted)	70
FVC (% predicted)	52
FEV$_1$/FVC	88%

What is the most likely cause given the results and clinical information?

Question 2

You are the junior doctor on the respiratory ward and have been asked to review the spirometry results of a 22-year-old student. He has been complaining of shortness of breath and a cough that wakes him from sleep. Spirometry was performed then repeated after administration of salbutamol. The results are shown below:

DOI: 10.1201/9781315113937-20

	RESULTS 1	RESULTS 2
FEV$_1$ (% predicted)	45	85
FVC (% predicted)	70	90
FEV$_1$/FVC	55	90

What is the most likely cause given the results and clinical information?

Question 3

You are the junior doctor on the respiratory ward and have been asked to review the spirometry results of a 67-year-old man. He is an ex-miner and has smoked for most of his life. Spirometry was performed then repeated after administration of salbutamol. The results are shown below:

	RESULTS 1	RESULTS 2
FEV$_1$ (% predicted)	40	42
FVC (% predicted)	65	68
FEV$_1$/FVC	55	56

What is the most likely cause given the results and clinical information?

SBAs

Question 1

1) Acute kidney injury
2) Asthma
3) COPD
4) Opiate overdose
5) Pulmonary embolism

You are the junior doctor in the ED and are asked to see a 45-year-old woman who was admitted short of breath. You take an ABG, the results of which are shown below:

	RESULTS
pH (NR: 7.35–7.45)	7.51
PaO$_2$ (NR: 11–13 kPa)	7.8 kPa
PaCO$_2$ (NR: 4.7–6.0 kPa)	3.9 kPa
HCO$_3$ (NR: 24–30 mmol/L)	21 mmol/L

What is the most likely diagnosis?

Question 2

1) Asthma
2) COPD
3) Diabetic ketoacidosis
4) Pulmonary embolism
5) Salicylate overdose

You are the junior doctor in the ED and are asked to see a 73-year-old man with shortness of breath. You take an ABG, the results of which are shown below:

	RESULTS
pH (NR: 7.35–7.45)	7.27
PaO$_2$ (NR: 11–13 kPa)	6.0
PaCO$_2$ (NR: 4.7–6.0 kPa)	8.1
HCO$_3$ (NR: 24–30 mmol/L)	32

What is the most likely diagnosis?

CHAPTER 2: RESPIRATORY INFECTION

EMQ 1:

1) Ciprofloxacin
2) Co-amoxiclav
3) Co-amoxiclav and intercostal drain
4) Doxycycline
5) Co-amoxiclav and clarithromycin IV
6) Meropenem
7) Oral amoxicillin
8) Oseltamivir
9) Piperacillin/tazobactam
10) Rest and paracetamol

For each of the following questions, please choose the most appropriate treatment. Each option may be used once, more than once, or not at all.

1. A 72-year-old female is admitted to hospital with a 3-day history of cough productive of purulent sputum, confusion and dyspnoea. Her observation chart records hypoxia, tachypnoea with a respiratory rate of 32 and hypotension with a blood pressure of 88 / 48. On auscultation of the chest, there are crackles at the left base with decreased chest expansion. The chest X-ray demonstrates consolidation at the left lower zone.

2. A 62-year-old male with a history of emphysema and type 2 diabetes mellitus sees his GP with a 4-day history of dry cough and shortness of breath proceeded by a sore throat. He has had several episodes of rigor at home. One

week ago he visited his grandchildren, who were suffering from symptoms of a "nasty cold". His GP notes his temperature to be $38.1^\circ C$ and sends him for a chest X-ray, which is normal.

3. A 92-year-old male is admitted from a nursing home with sudden onset over a day of breathlessness and cough productive of purulent sputum. He was noted to be vomiting the night before. His medical history includes a right middle cerebral artery territory stroke 2 years ago which has left him with residual left-sided weakness. On auscultation of his chest he has crepitations at the right base with reduced chest expansion. His chest X-ray shows consolidation at the right lower zone. The nurse mentions to you that the patient seemed to cough more when he was eating his lunch.

EMQ 2:

Options:

1) *Haemophilus influenzae*
2) Influenza A
3) Influenza C
4) *Legionella pneumophilia*
5) *Mycobacterium tuberculosis*
6) *Mycoplasma pneumoniae*
7) Respiratory syncytial virus (RSV)
8) *Staphylococcus aureus*
9) *Staphylococcus epidermis*
10) *Streptococcus pneumoniae*

For each of the following questions please select the organism or virus that you think is the single most likely cause of the patient's symptoms. Each option may be used once, more than once, or not at all.

1) A 58-year-old man presents with a history of high fever $(40.6^\circ C)$ and chills present over 24 hrs. He has developed a productive cough, chest pain and severe dyspnoea. On examination he appears unkempt with poor personal hygiene, smells strongly of alcohol and is cyanosed. There is dullness on percussion and bronchial breathing bilaterally, as well as a heart murmur. His chest X-ray shows bilateral multi-lobar consolidation and cavitation. He has no fixed abode and is currently in receipt of a regular methadone script.

2) A 35-year-old man presents to his GP with a worsening cough and chest pain that have developed over the past 10 days. He also reports a headache, sore throat and general malaise. On examination he has a fever $38.7^\circ C$ and generalised rhonchi with wheeze. There has been an unusual number of previously fit, young people turning up to surgery with similar symptoms over the last few months.

3) A 42-year-old woman presents with a gradual onset of fever, chills, a dry cough and general muscle pains over the last 3 days. On examination she seems generally unwell, is unstable on her feet and on auscultation there is bronchial breathing at both lung bases. She has just returned from a business conference, other attendees have reported similar symptoms.

SBAs respiratory infections:

For the following clinical scenarios please select the single most appropriate initial management:

Question 1

A 67-year-old woman presents with a productive cough and shortness of breath. Her vital signs are as follows: pulse 120 bpm, respiratory rate 32 per minute, BP 120/95 and a temperature of 38.5°C. On auscultation she has dullness to percussion and bronchial breathing at the right base.

1) Send home with no treatment
2) Prescribe a course of amoxicillin and get her GP to review in a week.
3) Insert a cannula into the second intercostal space mid-clavicular line.
4) Admit to hospital and start fluids and antibiotics.
5) Ask for a senior review and reserve a bed in ITU.

Question 2

A 6-year-old girl is brought into A&E. She looks very unwell, with a temperature of 39.4C, and is having difficulty breathing. She sits leaning forward with her mouth open, drooling, and she has a soft high-pitched stridor. Her parents say that she started complaining of a sore throat and developed a temperature about 6 hours previously.

1) Look in her eyes, ears and back of throat, to determine site of infection.
2) Insert a cannula and start IV antibiotics.
3) Give oral dexamethasone, oral prednisolone and nebulised budesonide.
4) Give oral dexamethasone, oral prednisolone and nebulised adrenaline.
5) Call an anaesthetist and senior paediatrician, to assess in Resus and facilitate rapid intubation of the patient.

Question 3

An 18-year-old female presents with shortness of breath, fever and cough productive of purulent sputum. Her symptoms are getting worse despite her GP starting a course of amoxicillin. She is normally fit and well. She has consolidation on her chest X-ray and you make a diagnosis of CAP. You have noticed an unusually high number of younger patients with pneumonia this year.
What is the most likely causative organism?

1. *Haemophilus influenzae*
2. *Legionella pneumophilia*
3. *Mycoplasma pneumonia*
4. *Staphylococcus aureus*
5. *Streptococcus pneumoniae*

CHAPTER 3: ASTHMA

EMQ

1. Home oxygen therapy
2. Montelukast
3. Omalizumab
4. Oral amoxicillin
5. Oral prednisolone
6. Refer to hospital for investigation
7. Salbutamol inhalers
8. Salbutamol nebulisers
9. Salmeterol
10. Theophylline

Question 1

Jamie is a 24-year-old engineer who has a long history of asthma. He currently takes salbutamol PRN and beclamethasone BD. Despite this, he is still bothered by a frequent chest tightness and shortness of breath necessitating use of his salbutamol inhaler. What will be your next step in managing him?

Question 2

Geoff is seen in the difficult asthma clinic at his local hospital because of frequent admissions with exacerbations of asthma. He has had 4 courses of oral steroids within 6 months. Which treatment may be considered next?

Question 3

Jim thinks he may have developed asthma because he has felt more short of breath and been coughing more than usual over the last few days. On auscultation, Jim has reduced air entry and bronchial breathing at the left base. He does not have a wheeze. How will you treat him?

SBAs:

Question 1

1. Which of these clinical features makes a diagnosis of asthma less likely (according to the BTS asthma guidelines)?
   1. Atopic disease in the family history.
   2. Dizziness.
   3. Previous diagnosis of eczema.
   4. Symptoms that worsen after taking propranolol.
   5. Wheeze.

Question 2

2. An 18-year-old student is brought to your ED acutely short of breath. Her respiratory rate is 30 and heart rate 115 beats per minute. She manages to perform a peak flow which is 200. Her SpO2 is 94% on air. On auscultation,

you hear a widespread expiratory wheeze throughout the lung fields. How will you manage this patient initially?

1. Administer salbutamol and ipratropium via an oxygen driven nebuliser.
2. Call ITU immediately.
3. Discharge with a course of oral steroids.
4. Give IV antibiotics.
5. Urgent needle decompression.

CHAPTER 4: CHRONIC OBSTRUCTIVE PULMONARY DISEASE

EMQ

1. Add a combination ICS/LABA inhaler.
2. Add salmeterol.
3. Add theophylline
4. Lung transplantation
5. Oral amoxicillin
6. Oral steroids.
7. Prescribe ipratropium
8. Prescribe salbutamol
9. Refer for LTOT.
10. Saline nebulisers

Question 1

1. Mr Cutler is a 68-year-old ex-foundry worker who has a history of increasing breathlessness. His history is suggestive of COPD. His FEV1 is 65%. He takes a SABA. What will be your next step in managing him?

Question 2

2. James has advanced COPD and is already taking with optimum inhaled therapy. His PaO_2 is 6.5kPa. He has noticed ankle swelling over the last few months.

Question 3

1. Mr Jefferson is taking a Ventolin inhaler. His most recent spirometry reveals his FEV1 is 48%. He is increasingly breathless. What will be your next step in managing him?

SBA

SBA: Question 1

1. Which of these investigation findings is not associated with COPD?
    1. A >400 mL improvement in FEV1 with inhaled salbutamol.
    2. A chest X-ray showing hyperinflation of the lungs.
    3. A full blood count showing a haemoglobin of 200g/l.

4. A reduced Tlco.
5. An FEV1/FVC ratio of < 0.7.

Question 2

2. Which of these is not an indication for starting LTOT?
    1. $PaO_2 < 7.3kPa$.
    2. $PaO_2 < 8kPa$ and nocturnal hypoxaemia.
    3. $PaO_2 < 8kPa$ and pulmonary hypertension.
    4. $PaO_2 < 8kPa$ and pulmonary oedema.
    5. $PaO_2 < 8kPa$ and secondary polycythaemia.

CHAPTER 5: LUNG MALIGNANCY

EMQ:

1) Cerebral metastases.
2) Hypercalcaemia.
3) Hypertrophic pulmonary osteoarthropathy.
4) Lambert-Eaton syndrome.
5) Lymphangitis carcinomatosa.
6) Neutropenic sepsis.
7) Spinal cord compression.
8) Superior vena cava obstruction.
9) Syndrome of inappropriate antidiuretic hormone.
10) Tumour lysis syndrome.

Question 1

A 59-year-old patient who smokes 60 cigarettes a day has recently been investigated for his cough and haemoptysis. His chest X-ray and CT showed spiculated lesions near the hilum, which he has been told are highly suggestive of cancer. When examining the samples taken during his bronchoscopy, the pathologist notes that there are "oat cells" present.

His vision has been deteriorating recently and he now struggles to read the paper. His wife notes that often he seems to have trouble saying what he wants to and gets frustrated; in addition he has had difficulty eating recently. However, he has come to see his GP because over the last couple of days he has collapsed a couple of times. On neurological examination of his lower limbs his GP notes decreased power. His wife reports that during these collapses he has lost consciousness, she has also noticed some brief jerking and on one occasion there was urinary incontinence.

Question 2

A 63-year-old who has been investigated for weight loss, clubbing and cough is diagnosed with lung cancer. Initially she reports having never smoked, but on further questioning admits being a social smoker at university.

The cancer is deemed to be inoperable but she is given a palliative course of chemotherapy. The patient has been complaining on bone pain since diagnosis, mostly in her hands and feet. On examination there is some swelling of her joints. She has also continued to lose weight and has had nausea and vomiting.

Question 3

A 73-year-old smoker who has been diagnosed with lung cancer comes into clinic. She has been getting progressively shorter of breath and is struggling to lay flat in bed at night. She reports struggling to deal with her diagnosis. However her sister who is with her is more hopeful, saying she looks a lot less gaunt than she did a few weeks ago

She has a past medical history of MI, breast cancer, hypertension and COPD. She reports drinking more heavily since her diagnosis.

You get the medical student to examine the patient. They note cachexia, clubbing and multiple spider naevi on the chest wall.

SBA

Question 1

Ahmed is a 38-year-old office worker, who comes in complaining of backache. He has lost 7 kg in the past 2 months. He also report that he has developed a cough and for the past couple of weeks he has been coughing up blood. He is usually fit and healthy, has no history of cardiac or respiratory disease and has never smoked. Despite being thin he appears to have some gynaecomastia on examination. The GP sends off a sputum sample looking for AFBs and sends him to the local hospital to have a CXR. The CXR shows multiple bilateral, suspicious spiculated masses. The radiologist diagnoses probable lung cancer on radiological appearance. The patient is booked for bronchoscopy to try and gain a histopathological diagnosis. What is the histopathology likely to show?

1) Adenocarcinoma.
2) Carcinoid tumour.
3) Metastatic lesion from a distant sight.
4) Small cell carcinoma.
5) Squamous cell carcinoma.

Question 2

Jane is a 59-year-old patient who was diagnosed with adenocarcinoma 2 years ago. It was picked up incidentally on a chest X-ray, which she had when she was planning a holiday to Australia. It was a single lesion, which was amenable to surgery; she had a lobectomy, pre-adjuvant and adjuvant chemotherapy, as well as post op radiotherapy. She is now being actively monitored for any relapse or emergence of distant metastases. Which scan would be best for this?

1) Chest + abdominal CT
2) Chest X-ray

3) Full-body MRI
4) Full skeletal survey
5) Pet-CT.

CHAPTER 6: PLEURAL DISEASE

EMQs

1. Cirrhosis
2. Empyema
3. Left ventricular failure
4. Lung malignancy
5. Meig's syndrome
6. Nephrotic syndrome
7. Pancreatitis
8. Parapneumonic effusion
9. Sarcoidosis
10. Tuberculosis

Question 1

You are the junior doctor on the respiratory ward and have been asked to see a 70-year old man who has been admitted via his GP. He is a vague historian and gives a history of shortness of breath which has been more noticeable over the last week or so. He mentions in passing that he's also been troubled by cough for the last 2 months and has coughed up blood "on occasion". He smoked for 50 years but gave up in his mid-sixties. On examination, he is apyrexial with dullness to percussion on the left side, associated with reduced air entry on auscultation. After confirming the presence of an effusion on chest X-ray, an aspirate is performed. The total protein is 36.1 g / L. What is the most likely cause of this patient's shortness of breath given the findings?

Question 2

You are the junior doctor on the respiratory ward and have been asked to see a 40-year-old man with shortness of breath who has been admitted via A&E. He is unkempt in appearance and reveals that he is homeless. He sleeps on the streets most nights but is occasionally able to secure a bed in a hostel. He gives a history of night sweats and claims to "cough up blood". His chest X-ray reveals a right-sided pleural effusion. The aspirate shows a protein content of 35.4 g / L; cytology reveals a high lymphocyte count; no bacteria are cultured after 48 hours. What is the most likely cause of this patient's shortness of breath given the findings?

Question 3

You are the junior doctor on the respiratory ward and have been asked to see a 75-year-old woman with a history of shortness of breath. Examination reveals dullness to percussion and crackles at both lung bases. The chest X-ray supports this, with bilateral pleural effusions and cardiomegaly. An aspirate is taken and protein content reported as 25.6 g / L. What is the most likely cause of this patient's shortness of breath given the findings?

SBA

Question 1

Jane has a history of asthma and has a presented to ED acutely short of breath. You performed a chest X-ray which revealed a 1.5cm left pneumothorax. There is no evidence of mediastinal shift. How do you proceed?

1. Admit for O2 and monitoring.
2. Arrange for chest drain insertion.
3. Aspirate with a 14G cannula.
4. Discharge with OPD review.
5. Perform an urgent needle decompression.

Question 2

An 18-year-old man experiences sudden onset of sharp chest pain whilst driving his car. The chest X-ray in ED shows a 1 cm pneumothorax. There is no associated shortness of breath and no previous history of respiratory disease. How do you proceed?

1. Admit for O2 and monitoring.
2. Arrange a VATS procedure.
3. Aspirate with a 14G cannula.
4. Discharge with OPD review
5. Refer for pleurodesis.

CHAPTER 7: PULMONARY EMBOLISM

EMQ

1. ABG
2. CTPA
3. CXR
4. D-dimer
5. ECG
6. Transthoracic echo
7. Thrombolysis
8. Thrombophilia screen
9. Unfractionated heparin
10. V/Q scan

Question 1

You are asked to review a patient in the ED who was admitted with shortness of breath and mild haemoptysis. She is a 38-year-old female who recently returned from New Zealand. She is 27 weeks pregnant. Her Wells score is calculated as 5.

What is the most appropriate action to perform next?

Question 2

You are asked to review a patient who has been admitted with shortness of breath and tachycardia. She was fit and well prior to admission with no recent surgery, immobility or long-haul flight. She denies leg swelling. Your consultant asks you to rule out PE given the sudden onset of symptoms, although he suspects an infection. Her Wells score is 1.5 .

What is the most appropriate action to perform next?

Question 3

You are asked to review a patient who has been admitted with acute shortness of breath. The CTPA reveals a large saddle embolus and the patient's systolic blood pressure is 82 mmHg.

What is the most appropriate action to perform next?

SBA

1. Apixaban for 3 months
2. Low-molecular-weight heparin for 3–6 months
3. Rivaroxaban for 6 months
4. Warfarin for 3 months, target INR 2.0 – 3.0
5. Warfarin for 6 months, target INR 2.0 – 3.0

Question 1

Mr Jones is admitted with acute shortness of breath. He is under the oncologist for colorectal cancer, currently undergoing chemotherapy. CTPA confirms pulmonary embolism. You start treatment with LMWH. What will be the ongoing management on discharge?

CHAPTER 8: TUBERCULOSIS

EMQ:

1) Bacterial pneumonia
2) B-cell lymphoma
3) Extra-pulmonary TB
4) Immune reconstitution inflammatory syndrome.
5) Latent TB
6) Lung cancer
7) MDR-TB
8) No disease process present
9) Pulmonary TB
10) Sarcoidosis
11) Wegner's granulomatosis

Question 1

Bill is referred to infectious diseases clinic to be tested for TB before starting TNF-α treatment for his rheumatoid arthritis. He has never had a BCG and denies chronic cough or interaction with anyone with TB previously. He confirms he has never had TB diagnosed in the past. His chest X-ray is normal and his tuberculin skin test is within normal limits. His IGRA is positive. Which of the above conditions is most likely to explain these test results?

Question 2

Dmitri is a 45-year-old homeless man. He is originally from Russia and has spent time incarcerated there. He smokes and is a heavy drinker. He has previously been treated for TB and is HIV positive, on anti-retrovirals. He comes into clinic after having been referred by his GP, for fever, night sweats and haemoptysis. His chest X-ray shows new cavitations and he is found to be sputum smear positive for acid fast bacilli. After 4 weeks of a DOTS regime he is still sputum smear positive, however he does report improvement in his symptoms.

Question 3

Daisy is a 23-year-old student. She was born in the UK, but had her BCG as a child. She comes to her GP complaining of fever, night sweats and weight loss. Her chest X-ray shows bilateral consolidation and hilar lymphadenopathy. She denies chronic cough or chest pain.

SBA

Question 1

Jetha is a 67-year-old man, he was born and brought up in India and moved to the UK in the 1980s. He has recently been diagnosed with TB, after complaining of a chronic cough and weight loss to his GP. His chest X-ray shows evidence of cavitating lesions and his sputum are positive for acid-fast bacilli. What drugs would his initial TB treatment regime consist of?

) Rifampicin and isoniazid.
2) Rifampicin, azithromycin, pyridoxine and ethambutol.
3) Rifampicin, isoniazid, pyrazinamide and erythromycin.
4) Rifampicin, isoniazid, pyrazinamide and ethambutol.
5) Rifampicin, isoniazid, pyridoxine and erythromycin.

Question 2

As mentioned in the previous question Jetha is sputum smear positive for acid-fast bacilli. What special measures will need to be taken in his treatment?

) Continue pyrazinamide for 4 months instead of 2.
2) In respiratory confinement for first 2 weeks of treatment.
3) No extra action needed. It's normal for a TB patient to be smear positive before treatment.
4) Repeat smear after 2 months, to check it's negative before continuation phase of treatment.
5) Send two further smears to confirm diagnosis.

CHAPTER 9: BRONCHIECTASIS AND CYSTIC FIBROSIS

EMQ: Cystic fibrosis inheritance

1. 1/2
2. 1/4
3. 1/8
4. 1/25
5. 1/100
6. 1/200
7. 1/250
8. 1/625
9. 1/1000
10. 1/2500

Question 1

Mr and Mrs Jones have a son with cystic fibrosis and are hoping to have a second child. They are concerned that this child may also be affected. What is the probability of them having a second child with cystic fibrosis?

Question 2

A woman is 8 weeks pregnant and known to be a carrier of cystic fibrosis.
   Her husband is Caucasian.
   What is the risk of the child having cystic fibrosis?

Question 3

A woman with cystic fibrosis attends for pre-pregnancy counselling. Her husband is known to be a carrier of cystic fibrosis.
   What is the risk of them having a child with CF?

SBA: COMPLICATIONS OF CYSTIC FIBROSIS

1. ABPA
2. Bronchiectasis
3. Non-tuberculous mycobacteria
4. Pneumothorax
5. *Pseudomonas aeruginosa* infection

David is a 21-year-old student with cystic fibrosis. His condition is normally very well controlled and he is very compliant with treatment. However, over the last few months he has suffered from a cough with purulent sputum and has noted some weight loss. FBC shows eosinophilia. A serum IgE is also elevated.
   Which of the above complications is most in keeping with this clinical picture?

SBA 1:

What is the most common cause of bronchiectasis in the developed world?

1) Alpha-1-antitrypsin deficiency
2) Cystic fibrosis
3) HIV/AIDS
4) Idiopathic pulmonary fibrosis
5) Rheumatoid arthritis

A 17-year-old patient has had recurrent respiratory tract infections since the age of 2 years. He presents complaining that he has had the same cough for the past 4 months, with fevers. He is coughing up mucopurulent sputum. He has intermittent haemoptysis, is becoming progressively shorter of breath, has wheeze and complains of being tired all the time. His girlfriend has just become pregnant and he would like to know if there is a chance his baby will have the same problems he's had. He can't remember the name of his diagnosis, but he's been told that his lungs are being damaged by repeated infections because of it.

The GP is not familiar with the patient's history and examines him. He has clubbing as well as widespread crackles, rhonchi and wheeze. On cardiac examination he struggles to hear the heart sounds clearly. What is the patient's diagnosis?

1) Cystic fibrosis
2) Immunoglobulin deficiency
3) Kartagener's syndrome
4) Prior childhood measles infection
5) Young's syndrome

CHAPTER 10: SARCOIDOSIS

EMQ:

1) Anterior uveitis
2) Acute closed-angle glaucoma
3) Haemoptysis: severe
4) Heerfordt syndrome
5) Myopathy
6) Neurosarcoidosis
7) Peripheral neuropathy
8) Pituitary infiltration
9) Pulmonary hypertension
10) TB

In each of the following scenarios, identify the complication of sarcoidosis that is most likely to have occurred in the patient described.

Question 1

Hope is a 35-year-old woman who has been diagnosed with sarcoidosis and is being treated with prednisolone due to failure of remission. She presents to her GP surgery with a severe headache and pain in her right eye. She complains of blurred vision and says that bright lights make her headache worse. When she is seen the GP notes that she has a red eye with a small fixed irregular pupil; small nodules on both irises are also observed.

Question 2

Chris is a 38-year-old man previously diagnosed with pulmonary sarcoidosis and is being followed up and observed. He had previously had a course of steroids. He complains of having had fevers and drenching night sweats for weeks, he has recently developed eye pain and now has blurred vision. His wife is with him and states that his face is looking more swollen and that he has been off his food recently. During the consultation you notice the patient is slurring and his face seems immobile. He has bilateral submandibular swelling, as well as swollen eyelids and inflamed eyes.

Question 3

A 40-year-old Russian man comes into respiratory clinic escorted by police. He is on leave from prison due to fevers, weight loss and a chronic cough. The police escorting him tell you that he has a string of criminal convictions in Russia also. They also admit that he has been coughing up blood recently. His chest X-ray shows some patchy infiltrates, hilar lymphadenopathy and distinct calcified lesions. He also has cervical lymphadenopathy.

SBA 1:

Which of the following rashes is most suggestive of a diagnosis of sarcoidosis?

1) Erythema migrans
2) Erythema nodosum
3) Maculopapular rash
4) Lupus pernio
5) Malar rash

SBA 2:

Which of the following signs would not be caused by systemic sarcoidosis?

1) Bilateral VII nerve palsy
2) Erythema nodosum
3) Hepatomegaly
4) Parotitis
5) Short PR interval on ECG

SBA 3:

You see a 40-year-old woman in a respiratory outpatient clinic. She was previously diagnosed with respiratory sarcoidosis and started on a course of steroids. You review her and she still complains of a dry cough and fatigue. Her chest X-ray shows bilateral lymphadenopathy. What stage is her respiratory disease?

1) 0
2) I
3) II
4) III
5) IV

CHAPTER 11: INTERSTITIAL LUNG DISEASE AND VASCULITIS

EMQ:

1) Ankylosing spondylitis
2) Caplan's syndrome
3) Dermatomyositis
4) Drug induced fibrosis
5) Extrinsic allergic alveolitis
6) Idiopathic pulmonary fibrosis
7) Lymphoid interstitial pneumonia
8) Sarcoidosis
9) Systemic lupus erythematosus
10) Systemic sclerosis

In each of the following questions, which is the most likely diagnosis?

Question 1

A 42-year-old woman comes into clinic complaining of fatigue. She has been suffering from fevers and weight loss over the last few months. She states that she has pains and aches all the time and that recently she has been having problems climbing the stairs and getting up from sitting. She also admits to mild breathlessness. When examining her you notice a purplish rash on her face, chest and on the back of her hands. She states that this is worsened when she has been outside for the day.

Question 2

A 55-year-old man comes in complaining of progressive breathlessness. His son had to take over the family farm a year ago, as he could no longer manage to run it. He admits to smoking in his 20s and 30s, but hasn't smoked since. He has been troubled by a cough, but isn't bringing any phlegm up. He remembers that his mother had a similar problem in her 60s and had to stop working. On examination he has clubbing and end inspiratory crackles bibasally.

Question 3

A 67-year-old woman with rheumatoid arthritis (RA) comes to see you in clinic. She complains of a dry cough and breathlessness, which have been getting worse over the last 12 months. Her husband was a smoker and a coal miner and died a few years previously. She is worried as she says that he suffered the same problems before he passed away. She states that she also used to smoke. You note that her RA has been well controlled for years with leflunomide and NSAIDS. Over the past couple of years she has been suffering with recurrent UTIs for which she has had multiple antibiotic courses and is now taking long term prophylactic trimethoprim.

EMQ:

1) Alpha-1-antitrypsin deficiency
2) Ankylosing spondylitis
3) Cystic fibrosis
4) Eosinophilic granulomatosis with polyangiitis (Churg-Strauss)
5) Goodpasture's syndrome
6) Granulomatosis with polyangiitis (Wegner's)
7) Idiopathic pulmonary fibrosis
8) Rheumatoid arthritis
9) Systemic lupus erythematosus
10) Young's syndrome

In each of the following questions which is the likely diagnosis?

Question 1

Jenny is a 40-year-old woman, who has been referred into respiratory clinic. She was diagnosed with asthma in her early 30s. However, her asthma has been difficult to control and the inhalers prescribed by her GP have been ineffective. She is referred in as she is complaining of becoming progressively wheezier and short of breath over the last few years. She also states that he has been coughing frequently and has been producing purulent sputum. On examination her chest is hyper-expanded with increased resonance on percussion and decreased breath sounds. Her chest X-ray shows basal bullae. Her routine bloods are normal other than an increased haematocrit and slightly deranged LFTs.

Question 2

John is a 52-year-old carpenter. He has spent his career building furniture and refurbishing old building. He comes into your practice complaining of increasing shortness of breath over the previous half a year. He complains that he is finding his job more difficult, he complains of fatigue, as well as muscular and joint pains that have developed over the same period. On further questioning he admits to having lost 5 kg over the last 3 months and has had recurrent fevers. He is very concerned as he remembers his father and grandfather died in their

50s after having a similar period of illness. He can't recall what the illness his father had. On examination he has bibasal fine crepitations and clubbing.

Question 3

Niall is a 28-year-old man. He is a smoker and has recently been diagnosed with high blood pressure, for which he is currently being investigated. He has been suffering from fever and chills recently. He complains that he is struggling to play tennis for his local team because of joint pains and fatigue, as well as shortness of breath. He also states that he has had a cough over the last 3 weeks and has finally come into the doctors as a few days ago he started coughing up blood. He also admits that he has had a couple of cases of bloody urine recently. He states that he has put off coming to the doctors as he is afraid that he has cancer due to this smoking.

SBA 1:

A 53-year-old woman comes into her GP surgery with progressive shortness of breath. Her past medical history includes hypothyroidism and GORD: she is currently taking levothyroxine and omeprazole. She presented a few months ago with Raynaud's phenomenon and she states this has worsened. On examination you notice the skin on her hands is tight and shiny, and on auscultation of the chest you hear fine end-inspiratory crackles. What antibody would be most helpful in this patient's diagnosis?

1) Anti-centromere antibody (ACA)
2) Anti-double stranded DNA antibody (anti-dsDNA)
3) Anti-neutrophil cytoplasmic antibody (ANCA)
4) Anti-nuclear antibody (ANA)
5) Anti-topoisomerase-1 antibody (anti-Scl 70)

SBA 2:

Which of the following drugs is most associated with pulmonary fibrosis as a side effect?

1) Azathioprine
2) Bleomycin
3) Ciclosporin
4) Cyclophosphamide
5) Trimethoprim

SBA 3:

Terry is a 32-year-old who presents to his GP with a history of cough, shortness and haemoptysis. He says that over the last month or so his asthma has been getting worse and that he has needed to use his Ventolin inhaler. He says that he has suffered from asthma, hay fever and sinus problems since he was a child. As well as this, he says that he gets recurrent nose bleeds that he finds embarrassing and inconvenient.

He also describes suffering from muscular pains and general malaise and you notice that he has a strange rash on his hands. He has never smoked, he was born and raised in the UK and has never travelled abroad. The GP does an FBC and a chest X-ray. When the results come back the bloods show eosinophilia and the chest X-ray has bilateral infiltrates. What is the likely diagnosis?

1) Eosinophilic granulomatosis with polyangiitis
2) Goodpasture's syndrome
3) Granulomatosis with polyangiitis
4) Systemic lupus erythematosus
5) Tuberculosis

CHAPTER 12: PULMONARY HYPERTENSION

EMQ:

1) Balloon atrial septostomy
2) Bosentan
3) Carvedilol
4) Diltiazem
5) Epoprostenol
6) Exercise
7) Influenza and pneumococcal vaccinations.
8) Sildenafil
9) Transplantation (Allogenic)
10) Transplantation (Xenogenic)

In each of the following cases, please select the next most appropriate step in treatment of the patient's PH:

Question 1

A 62-year-old Ugandan man comes into the respiratory clinic with progressive shortness of breath and chest pain on exertion. He has no previous history of cardiac or respiratory diseases. He has never smoked and only drinks occasionally. On examination he has swelling and abdominal distension that has developed over the last month. His BP is 130/85 and all of the blood tests that you have requested have come back as normal. The only previous radiological finding of significance is incidental bladder calcification on an abdominal X-ray. An ECG and echocardiogram are performed which show right ventricular hypertrophy, but no evidence of ischaemic disease. Pulmonary hypertension is suspected so a right heart catheter is done; mean pulmonary artery pressure is 32 mmHg, this decreases to 22 mmHg after IV infusion of epoprostenol.

Question 2

A 57-year-old man comes into respiratory clinic with progressive shortness of breath and chest pain on exercise. He has no previous history of respiratory diseases, but reports having had rheumatic fever in his early 20s. He has never smoked and drinks only occasionally. On examination he has swelling and abdominal distension that has developed over the last month. His BP is 190/105 and all of the blood tests that you have requested have come back as normal. On auscultation of his chest you hear a mid-diastolic rumbling murmur. An ECG and echocardiogram are performed which show right and left ventricular hypertrophy, as well as mitral valve stenosis but no evidence of ischaemic disease. Pulmonary hypertension is suspected so a right heart catheter is done; he is diagnosed with WHO group II PH, with a mean pulmonary artery pressure of is 32 mmHg, which does not decrease after an IV infusion of epoprostenol.

Question 3

A 52-year-old woman who has previously been diagnosed with pulmonary hypertension with multiple PEs. Previous echocardiograms have all demonstrated right ventricular hypertrophy and left-to-right flow between the atria which is thought to be a normal variant. When you follow her up in clinic she reports being very short of breath at rest, despite being on multiple vasodilatory medications. On examination she is obviously distressed and breathless at rest. She has clubbing, as well as a bluish tinge in her fingers around her mouth and under her tongue. She has crepitations in both lung fields. When you check the report of her repeat echo today, it states that there is again intra-atrial flow which is from right to left.

SBA 1:

What mean pulmonary artery pressure (mmHg) is the threshold for diagnosing pulmonary hypertension (PH)?

) 8
) 15
) 21
) 25
) 30

SBA 2:

Which of the following findings would you expect to find when examining the JVP of a patient with PH?

) Cannon a wave
) Elevated JVP with a large a wave

3) Kussmaul's sign
4) Non-pulsatile elevated JVP
5) Absent x descent

CHAPTER 13: FUNGAL DISEASES OF THE LUNG

EMQ:

1) Broncho-alveolar lavage
2) Chest X-ray
3) Chest HRCT
4) Differentiated WCC
5) Enzyme immunoassay
6) HIV-1 + 2 antibodies
7) MRI head
8) Serum LDH
9) Sputum smear and culture
10) VATS + biopsy, culture and staining

Question 1

An HIV-positive patient presents to hospital with cough, fever and shortness of breath. It is noted by the ID registrar that she hasn't attended HIV clinic or collected his prescriptions for anti-retrovirals in the last year. She desaturates during exercise and a chest X-ray shows bilateral peri-hilar opacities. An induced sputum sample is PAS (periodic acid-Schiff) staining is carried out; this shows cysts resembling crushed ping pong balls and foamy alveolar macrophages.

Question 2

A patient with a history of asthma presents to the hospital respiratory outpatient clinic. He has a history of fever, weight loss, chest pain, purulent cough and progressively worsening wheeze. After initial investigations respiratory consultant suspects invasive bronchopulmonary aspergillosis. What would be the gold standard investigation for confirming the diagnosis?

Question 3

A patient previously unknown to services presents to hospital. He gives a history of cough, fever and shortness of breath. He is reticent to give further history, but appears emaciated and has track marks on his arms. He desaturates during exercise and a chest X-ray shows bilateral peri-hilar opacities. An induced sputum sample is PAS (periodic acid-Schiff) staining is carried out; this shows clumps resembling crushed "ping pong balls", typical of *P. jirovecii*. What further investigation should be done at this point?

SBA 1:

What is the prevalence of allergic bronchopulmonary aspergillosis in the cystic fibrosis population?

) 2%

) 5%

) 10%

) 15%

) 20%

SBA 2:

A mycetoma is found incidentally on a patient's chest X-ray. The patient had previously been treated for pulmonary TB 4 years ago. The patient is asymptomatic and healthy, what is the best initial treatment in this case?

) Itraconazole 200 mg PO BD

) Ketoconazole 200 mg PO OD

) No treatment required

) Surgical removal

) Voriconazole 6 mg/kg IV BD

CHAPTER 14: SLEEP DISORDERED BREATHING

SBA 1:

Which of the following clinical tools is used to diagnose obstructive sleep apnoea?

) Epworth sleepiness scale

) Polysomnography

) Nasolaryngoscopy

) Sleep study

) Pulse oximetry

SBA 2:

What is the strongest risk factor for developing OSAHS?

) Family history

) High alcohol intake

) Male gender

) Obesity

) Smoking

CHAPTER 15: OCCUPATIONAL LUNG DISEASE

SBA 1:

A woman comes into her GP on Monday morning complaining that she has been suffering from wheeze and breathlessness, for a few months. She has taken a day off working as a scrub nurse at the local hospital to come and see you. There has been extensive building works going on in her department and feels that the dust from this is causing her symptoms. She describes becoming wheezy towards the evening; she also describes a recurring itchy rash on both of her hands. You examine her and find no rash and her chest is clear bilaterally with no wheeze. She has no past history of respiratory problems and doesn't smoke. What is the likely cause of her problems

1) Asbestos
2) Chlorhexidine
3) Food allergens
4) Latex
5) Malingering

SBA 2:

What risk factor most increases the chance of a patient with asbestosis developing mesothelioma?

1) Asbestos exposure for >15 years
2) BAP-1 gene mutation
3) High number of pleural plaques on chest X-ray
4) Lifelong smoker
5) Previous infection with simian virus-40

CHAPTER 16: RESPIRATORY EMERGENCIES

EMQ: Immediate management of respiratory distress

1. 15L O_2 via non re-breathe mask IM adrenaline, IV hydrocortisone.
2. 15L O_2 via non re-breathe mask nebulised salbutamol and ipratropium, IV hydrocortisone.
3. 15L O_2 via non re-breathe mask, IV fluid bolus, IV heparin.
4. Chest drain insertion
5. Continuous positive airway pressure (CPAP).
6. Discuss with senior regarding commencing IV magnesium sulphate.
7. Discuss with ITU regarding intubation and ventilation
8. Non invasive ventilation (NIV).
9. Oxygen titrated to ABG results, salbutamol and ipratropium nebs, PO prednisolone
10. Urgent needle decompression.

Question 1

A 65-year-old lifelong smoker present with shortness of breath, productive cough and wheeze. He is using his accessory muscles and pursing his lips to breathe.

Question 2

A 17-year-old girl presents with shortness of breath, wheeze and facial swelling.

Question 3

A 36-year-old man is involved in a road traffic accident. He develops acute shortness of breath. On examination you noted resonance to percussion on the left side and deviation of the trachea towards the right.

SBAs

1. Angiography and embolisation
2. High-dose dexamethasone
3. Nebulised salbutamol
4. Oral prednisolone
5. Thrombolysis

Question 1

A 78-year-old gentleman is admitted with shortness of breath. He has a 40 pack-year smoking history and has been troubled by a cough for the last 3 months. During the consultation, you note that his face and arms appear swollen and he is plethoric. On examination, he has a non-pulsatile raised JVP. What is the most appropriate immediate management?

CHAPTER 17: SMOKING AND THE LUNG

SBA 1:

What is the quit rate for a patient who uses the NHS stop smoking service, after 1 year?

a) 1%
b) 4%
c) 10%
d) 15%
e) 25%

SBA 2:

If you were working in a NHS stop smoking service which prescribed varenicline, which of the following patients would it be inappropriate to prescribe this medication to?

1) 28-year-old male has completed a 12-week course of varenicline and has remained abstinent. However he requests further treatment as he still has strong urges to smoke.
2) A 30-year-old man has tried nicotine replacement therapy previously and has failed to quit. He was hospitalised as a child because of meningitis and has been told by his parents that he had seizures during hospitalisation. These have not recurred.
3) 32-year-old woman smokes 20 cigarettes a day and expresses a wish to quit smoking. She had asthma as a child but otherwise has no PMH and is fit and well. She admits to needing counselling and treatment previously for self-harming.
4) A 60-year-old man with a history of ischaemic heart disease and COPD wants to quit.
5) A 64-year-old woman has been diagnosed with lung cancer. She states that she would like to quit smoking.

Answers

CHAPTER 1: CLINICAL ASSESSMENT

EMQ: Lung function test

Question 1

Answer: **Drug-induced pulmonary fibrosis**

The spirometry results reveal a restrictive pattern (reduced FVC and preserved FEV_1/FVC). This suggests a fibrotic lung disease. Rheumatoid arthritis is associated with pulmonary fibrosis in itself, although this is not an answer on the list of possible options. The drug history is the giveaway in this case: pulmonary fibrosis is a potential side effect of the disease modifying anti-rheumatic drug methotrexate, which is commonly prescribed in RA.

Question 2

Answer: **Asthma**

This is an obstructive spirometry pattern associated with reversibility upon administration of a β_2-agonist. This is strongly suggestive of asthma, which is supported by the patient's young age and morning symptoms.

Question 3
Answer: **COPD**

The spirometry results show a reduced FEV$_1$ and FVC as well as a reduced FEV$_1$/FVC ratio. This is typical of an obstructive pattern. Unlike the previous case, this one shows no reversibility with salbutamol. This in combination with the patient's age and smoking history makes COPD the most likely diagnosis.
ABG SBAs

SBAs

Question 1
Answer: **PE**

The first thing to comment on is the PaO$_2$ which is clearly low. The PaCO$_2$ is also low, so this is a type 1 respiratory failure. The pH of 7.51 is alkalotic and the low PaCO$_2$ means that this is a respiratory alkalosis, which tends to be due to excessive ventilation. There is a small degree of renal compensation as evidenced by the low HCO$_3$. Of the 5 causes listed, PE is the most likely cause: this causes a V/Q mismatch which results in type 1 respiratory failure and compensatory hyperventilation, which in turn reduces the PaCO$_2$ and causes an alkalotic picture.

Question 2
Answer: **COPD**

Again, begin by commenting on the PaO$_2$. In this patient, it is low. The PaCO$_2$ is raised, so this is a type 2 respiratory failure. The low pH and high CO$_2$ correspond with a respiratory acidosis. The raised bicarbonate level indicates an attempt by the kidneys to compensate, which is insufficient. It is also worth noting that renal compensation does not occur in the acute stages and is therefore suggestive of a chronic disease process. This picture might be seen in COPD and if this was an ABG taken during a period of stability in the patient's disease, it might be an indication for LTOT.

CHAPTER 2: RESPIRATORY INFECTION

Answers EMQ 1:

1. Answer: **IV Co-amoxiclav and clarithromycin**
   This patient has severe community-acquired pneumonia. She has clinical signs of pneumonia, and her chest X-ray shows consolidation. Her CURB-65 score is 4 (confusion, respiratory rate >30, systolic BP <90, >65 years old), and she should therefore be treated with IV co-amoxiclav and clarithromycin. Amoxicillin, doxycycline or co-amoxiclav alone would not provide- a broad enough spectrum. If this patient failed to respond to initial therapy she should be referred to critical care.

2. Answer: **Oseltamivir**

This patient has presented with symptoms typical of influenza. He had respiratory symptoms proceeded by a coryzal illness and has recently had contact with others suffering from respiratory viral illness. He has a non-productive cough, and his chest X-ray is normal which goes against diagnosis of pneumonia. His pre-existing chest disease and diabetes mellitus puts him in the high-risk group so he should receive oseltamivir. He should also be offered an annual influenza vaccine, and be advised on simple management-rest, fluids and paracetamol.

3. Answer: **Co-amoxiclav**

This patient has an aspiration pneumonia. His previous stroke is a risk factor for aspiration, and the nursing staff on the ward have alerted you to the fact that he may have dysphagia. Aspiration pneumonia will typically develop in the right lower lobe, as the right bronchus is more vertical than the left (because of this, inhaled foreign objects will more often go down the right bronchus than the left). Co-amoxiclav provides adequate spectrum cover as a first line antibiotic.

Answers EMQ 2:

1) Answer: ***Staphylococcus aureus***

Homelessness, alcoholism, intravenous drug use and valvular disease are all risk factors for developing *S. aureus* pneumonia. The high temperature and the cavitating legions on X-ray are typical of this organism. Also the speed of onset and the seriousness of the symptoms suggest *S. aureus*. Although other organisms can cause a similar clinical picture the onset is generally more insidious. A heart murmur could also suggest he has developed infective endocarditis, which with *S. aureus* as the infective agent may progress rapidly.

2) Answer: ***Mycoplasma pneumoniae***

The pneumonia is in a previously fit and well young adult with no risk factors. This, along with as a slow onset and relatively mild symptomology suggests *M. pneumoniae*. The description of the outbreak among young adults is also characteristic.

3) Answer: ***Legionella pneumophilia*** (**Legionnaires' disease**)

The clinical picture could suggest either Influenza A or *L. pneumophilia*. However, ataxia is a characteristic finding in Legionnaires' disease, whereas it does not occur in influenza. *Legionella pneumophilia* survives in humidified water and is transmitted via the aerosolised water particles. In this case the patient has probably been infected via hotel air-conditioning units.

SBAs respiratory infections:

Question 1 – Answer

Admit to hospital and start fluids and antibiotics.

The clinical picture for this patient suggests that she has pneumonia. A urea is not yet available for this patient, but she has a CURB − 65 score of at least 2 and she is tachycardic. Doing a blood test and obtaining a urea as well as measuring O_2 sats would be useful to help further decisions on management. Her mortality risk with a CURB score of 2 is 3 − 15%. She will need antibiotics; her tachycardia suggests she would likely need fluids as well. NICE guidelines suggest that patients with CURB – 65 scores ³2 should be considered for hospital admission and if ³3 are considered for ITU. This patient may need ITU in future, but the initial most appropriate management is to start treatment and to arrange for hospital admission.

Question 2 – Answer

Call an anaesthetist and senior paediatrician, to assess in Resus and facilitate rapid intubation of the patient.

The most likely diagnosis here is epiglottitis (most likely bacterial). This is suggested by her having to lean forward to maintain her airway, the soft high-pitched stridor and drooling (suggesting an inability to swallow her saliva); her epiglottis is swollen, and her airway is compromised. It would be important not to distress the patient or examine the back of her throat without an anaesthetist present as it is likely to cause spasm and airway obstruction. Initially the most important thing is to move the patient to Resus and have an anaesthetist to intubate the child if needed. After this, high-flow oxygen and adrenaline are sometimes given if there is delay in an anaesthetist arriving.

Question 3 – Answer

Mycoplasma pneumonia

Although *S. pneumoniae* is the most common pathogen in community acquired pneumonia, this patient has not improved despite amoxicillin. *M. pneumonia* occurs in outbreaks amongst young patients every few years. She does not have any underlying chest disease which makes *H. influenzae* less likely, and has no risk factors for *S. aureus*. Patients with *L. pneumophilia* infection are typically more unwell.

CHAPTER 3: ASTHMA

EMQ

Question 1

Answer: **Salmeterol**

This patient is already on a short-acting beta agonist and inhaled corticosteroids. This is step 2 of the BTS stepwise management of asthma. According to the BTS guidelines, the next step would be to add a long-acting beta agonist e.g. salmeterol. You would also consider increasing the dose of beclamethasone as part of stage 3 of the BTS guidelines.

Question 2

Answer: **Omalizumab**

Omalizumab may be indicated in this case, provided this patient has been managed, and is compliant with, the first 4 stages of the BTS stepwise approach. Omalizumab is licensed for use in patients with at least 2 exacerbations requiring hospital admission within the last year, or 3 exacerbations of which one required hospital admission and the other 2 required increased treatment and monitoring e.g. in ED. Patients should also have confirmation of an IgE-mediated allergy to a perennial allergen. It is discontinued if there is no response within 16 weeks of starting treatment.

Question 3

Answer: **Oral amoxicillin**

This history is not suggestive of asthma. Clinical examination does not reveal a wheeze and the onset is too acute. The findings on auscultation suggest that this patient may have a lower respiratory tract infection, for which amoxicillin is the first-line treatment. If he continues to have symptoms after the infection is treated and the GP has a clinical suspicion of asthma, a trial of inhaled salbutamol may be appropriate.

SBAs:

Question 1

Answer: **Dizziness**

Dizziness is not a typical feature of asthma, whereas all of the other options listed could potentially be found in an asthmatic patient.

Question 2

Answer: **Administer salbutamol and ipratropium via and oxygen driven nebuliser**

This is an acute severe asthma exacerbation (HR > 110 bpm, RR > 25 but $SpO_2 > 92\%$). It would not be appropriate to discharge her with oral steroids given the severity of her symptoms. There is no evidence of infection, so antibiotics are not indicated. You should administer salbutamol and ipratropium via an oxygen driven nebuliser in the first instance. In addition, steroids (IV or oral) should be given. You do not need to call ITU for this patient at present but would consider this if she failed to improve with therapy or developed life-threatening features. There is no role for needle decompression in acute severe asthma.

CHAPTER 4: CHRONIC OBSTRUCTIVE PULMONARY DISEASE

EMQ

Question 1
Answer: **Add salmeterol**

According to the NICE guidelines for management of COPD, the next step following either a SABA or SAMA for a patient with an FEV_1 of > 50% is to add either a LAMA (such as tiotropium bromide) or LABA (such as salmeterol).

Question 2
Answer: **Refer for LTOT**

This patient is eligible for LTOT as his PaO_2 is less than 7.3kPa and he has peripheral oedema. The criteria are:
- PaO_2 < 7.3kPa *or*
- PaO_2 < 8kPa *and*
  - Nocturnal hypoxaemia
  - Peripheral oedema
  - Secondary polycythaemia
  - Pulmonary hypertension.

Question 3
Answer: **Add a combination ICS/LABA inhaler**

According to the NICE guidelines for management of COPD, the next step following either a SABA or SAMA for a patient with an FEV_1 of < 50% is to add either a LAMA (e.g. tiotropium) or a combination ICS/LABA inhaler such as Seretide (salmeterol and beclamethasone) or Symbicort (formoterol and budesonide).

SBA

SBA: Question 1
Answer: **A > 400ml improvement in FEV1 with inhaled salbutamol**

An improvement of > 400ml or > 15% with inhaled salbutamol would be more suggestive of a diagnosis of asthma. The other findings may be seen in COPD, although the chest X-ray changes and polycythaemia might not be seen in the early stages of the disease and a reduced Tlco is not specific for COPD.

Question 2

Answer: **PaO$_2$ < 8kPa and pulmonary oedema**

This is the only incorrect option on the list. PaO$_2$ < 8kPa and *peripheral* oedema is an indication for LTOT but pulmonary oedema is not.

NICE states that people receiving LTOT should breathe supplemental oxygen for at least 15 hours a day. If they smoke, it is important to warn them about the risk of fire and explosion.

CHAPTER 5: LUNG MALIGNANCY

EMQ:

Answers

Question 1: **Lambert-Eaton syndrome:** The symptoms alluded to in the history would be typical of Lambert-Eaton syndrome. He is having difficulty reading due to his diplopia. His difficulty speaking is due to dysarthria (although the description by his wife is ambiguous). His difficulty eating will be caused by both dysphagia and dry mouth. He has weakness as noted by the GP when he does a neurological examination. His collapses are due to orthostatic hypotension; they are vaso-vagal collapses. It is worth noting that some jerking on passing out and urinary incontinence is relatively common in vaso-vagal syncope (as opposed to the sustained rhythmical jerking of epilepsy).

The histological observations of the pathologist confirm SCLC, the lung cancer type responsible for this autoimmune, neuromuscular condition.

The lack of a headache, nausea and vomiting, as well as the lack of neuroanatomical consistency, makes cerebral metastases very unlikely. On top of this, as mentioned previously, he is having vaso-vagal syncope rather than fits. Although he has leg weakness, the rest of the clinical picture does not fit with spinal cord compression.

Question 2: **Hypertrophic pulmonary osteoarthropathy:** The patient has the classic triad of clubbing, joint pain and joint swelling. The nausea and vomiting is a red herring: it is mentioned in the question that the patient has started chemotherapy; this is a very common side effect of this treatment.

Her smoking story would be very typical of a patient with adenocarcinoma of the lung, which is the lesion that is associated with HPOA.

Question 3: **Superior vena cava obstruction:** This woman has dyspnoea and orthopnoea. Her sister mistakenly thinks she has put weight back on, as her face is less gaunt (facial swelling). The medical student confirms that in fact she is cachectic, he also mistakenly notes spider naevi; these are in fact dilated veins across her chest wall due to venous congestion secondary to tumour obstruction.

Lymphangitis carcinomatosa would be an explanation of progressive breathlessness, if this was a metastatic relapse from her previous breast cancer. However, it would be less likely and it doesn't fully explain the clinical picture.

SBA

Answer

The answer is B. Although adenocarcinoma is the most common histological group of primary lung cancers, metastatic disease in the lung is more common still. The radiological appearance is also suggestive of metastases, as the lesions in lung are multiple and bilateral. Adenocarcinoma would usually present radiologically as a single peripheral lung lesion. The fact that the patient has never smoked makes primary lung cancer at this age unlikely (this would be a young patient to develop lung cancer even if he did smoke). The gynaecomastia might be a clue as to his primary lesion being testicular cancer, as a raised B-HCG would cause this. The back pain could be from working a computer all day, or could be another site of metastases.

Answer

The answer is E. PET-CT is the best modality for identifying local recurrence and distant metastases; indeed it is the only one that would detect micrometastases. Chest X-ray is not sensitive enough and would not identify distant recurrence. MRI and skeletal survey are inappropriate. Chest and abdominal CT would be inferior.

CHAPTER 6: PLEURAL DISEASE

EMQs

Question 1

Answer: **Lung malignancy**

This effusion is exudative in nature. The differential for exudative effusions includes bronchial malignancy, infections and PE. The patient reports a chronic cough, associated with haemoptysis. This in itself should be enough to raise suspicions of lung cancer and in combination with the age and smoking history of this patient, you would be highly suspicious of malignancy.

Question 2

Answer: **Tuberculosis**

The effusion is exudative and the causes of an effusion of this type include bronchial malignancy, infections and PE. All of these are associated with haemoptysis. Failure to culture bacteria makes a simple pneumonia less probable. The diagnosis of TB is supported by the high lymphocyte count, history of night sweats and the patient's social history: homelessness is a risk factor for development of TB. You would need to send the aspirate for microscopy for acid-fast bacilli and culture on Lowenstein-Jensen medium.

Question 3

Answer: **Left ventricular failure**

The protein content of this effusion is <30 g/L which means it is transudative in nature. Causes of transudative effusions include nephrotic syndrome, cirrhosis, hypoalbuminaemia and cardiac failure. The chest X-ray findings of bilateral effusions with cardiomegaly mean that cardiac failure is the most likely explanation in this case. You would also want to enquire about symptoms of orthopnoea (breathlessness when lying flat) and paroxysmal nocturnal dyspnoea (waking up breathless in the night) to support this diagnosis, as well as establishing the patient's past history of cardiac disease.

SBA

Question 1

Answer: **Arrange for chest drain insertion.**

This patient is symptomatic has a pre-existing respiratory disease – a high-risk feature according to the BTS guidelines for pneumothorax. She should have a chest drain inserted under radiological guidance and be admitted to hospital. As there is no evidence of mediastinal shift then the pneumothorax is not under tension and urgent needle decompression would be inappropriate. A symptomatic pneumothorax of this size without high-risk characteristics may be initially managed with aspiration using a 14G cannula.

Question 2

Answer: **Discharge with OPD review.**

This patient has no respiratory history so this is a primary spontaneous pneumothorax. As there is no dyspnoea, the BTS guidelines recommend discharge home with outpatient follow-up every 2–4 days. Procedures such as VATS or pleurodesis may be appropriate in those presenting with a second pneumothorax.

CHAPTER 7: PULMONARY EMBOLISM

EMQ

Question 1

Answer: **V/Q scan**

The Wells score of 5 indicated a high probability of PE. Under normal circumstances a CTPA would be the next course of action, but in this case the patient's pregnancy means that the radiation dose would be unacceptable. A V/Q scan is preferable in this case. If there was to be an undue delay, then it would be reasonable to begin a heparin infusion whilst waiting for the scan.

Question 2

Answer: **D-dimer**

Her Wells score and clinical history make PE less probable than in the previous case. A D-dimer is a useful investigation to perform in this case, as a negative result excludes PE. A positive result would necessitate further investigation e.g. CTPA.

Question 3

Answer: **Thrombolysis**

In patients with a PE and systolic BP < 90mmHg , thrombolysis should be considered. This would be administered by a senior doctor in a monitored environment, only if there were no contraindications (e.g. bleeding risk).

SBA

Answer: **Low-molecular-weight heparin for 3–6 months**

As this patient has a known history of malignancy, he should be treated with LMWH as per the NICE guidelines for 3–6 months. Following this, lifelong oral anticoagulation should be commenced.

CHAPTER 8: TUBERCULOSIS

EMQ:

Answers

Question 1: Latent TB. There is no evidence of active infection and no past history of TB infection, as demonstrated by the chest X-ray and the negative TST. The patient has no active symptoms. The lack of BCG might put him at greater risk of acquiring TB if he lives in a community with high prevalence. His positive IGRA demonstrates that he has been infected with TB at some point previously, the lack of PMH suggests that his infection is latent.

Question 2: MDR-TB. The patient is still smear positive for AFBs after a month of DOTS treatment. The fact he has been treated previously, possibly unsuccessfully, and his HIV put him at greater risk of developing MDR-TB. As does his past background.

NB. MDR-TB is more highly prevalent in Russia. It is especially common in the prison population.

Question 3: B-cell lymphoma. The patient is in an age group when this disease is prevalent. She has no risk factors for TB and the symptomology doesn't fit with this. The chest X-ray findings would also be more typical of lymphoma than TB.

SBA

Question 1

Answer: D. A quadruple therapy is needed in the initial stages of treating TB. An easy way to remember this is with the pneumonic RIPE. Pyridoxine is vitamin B6 and is given if the patient is at risk of peripheral neuropathy; it is given in addition to the four TB drugs if required. Erythromycin and azithromycin are not first-line TB drugs.

Question 2

Answer: B. The patient will need to be kept in Respiratory confinement until 2 weeks of treatment are completed (or until three consecutive smears are negative) as per NICE guidelines. Ideally this would be in a hospital negative pressure side room. The patient is an infection risk to others because his positive smear indicates a high bacterial load and that he is aerosolising those bacteria. Contacts that are living with the patient will require post-exposure prophylaxis.

CHAPTER 9: BRONCHIECTASIS AND CYSTIC FIBROSIS

EMQ:

Question 1
Answer: **1/4**
Cystic fibrosis is inherited in an autosomal recessive fashion. Thus when two carriers have a child, there is a 1/4 chance of them being affected, a 1/2 chance of them carrying the gene and a 1/4 chance of being unaffected and not carrying the gene. 1/25 is the carrier frequency in the Caucasian population and 1/2500 is the proportion of affected individuals within the Caucasian population.

Question 2
Answer: **1/100**
There is a 1/25 chance her husband is carrier. There is a 1/1 chance the woman herself is a carrier, meaning a 1/25 chance that both are carriers.

Multiplied by 1/4 (the chance that the two carriers with have an affected child), this comes to 1/100 .

Question 3

Answer: **1/2**

The woman in this scenario has two mutated recessive genes for CF; the man has one mutated gene and one not mutated. There is a 1/2 chance that the abnormal gene will be passed on by the father. There is a 1/1 chance that the mother will pass on the abnormal gene and a 1/2 overall risk of the child having CF.

SBA: COMPLICATIONS OF CYSTIC FIBROSIS

Answer: **ABPA**

ABPA, bronchiectasis, NTM and *Pseudomonas* infection could all contribute to the cough and purulent sputum. However, eosinophilia and raised IgE are most suggestive of ABPA.

SBA 1:

Answer: B. Cystic fibrosis is the most common cause of bronchiectasis in the developed world.

Answer: C. The patient is suffering from bronchiectasis because of damage from recurrent infections due to cilia dysmotility. The reason the GP struggles to hear his heart sound is because of his dextrocardia, which is pathognomonic. The fact that he naturally impregnated his girlfriend also rules out the more common childhood cause of bronchiectasis: cystic fibrosis and also Young's syndrome.

CHAPTER 10: SARCOIDOSIS

EMQ:

Answers

Question 1: **Anterior uveitis.**

The fact that the pupil is small and irregular would be suggestive of anterior uveitis. The nodules on the irises are Busacca nodules and are typical in granulomatous forms of anterior uveitis such as sarcoidosis.

Acute closed-angle glaucoma would more typically have a fixed and dilated pupil with a hazy cornea. Extensive infiltration of the pituitary might cause a visual defect (e.g. bitemporal hemianopia) due to pressure on the optic chiasm. It could also cause SUNCT headaches, which would present as a red and weeping eye, however there would be no pupil abnormality.

Question 2: Heerfordt's syndrome.

This is a syndromic presentation of sarcoidosis, which includes:

- Chronic fevers
- Parotid swelling (painless)
- Uveitis
- VII nerve palsy.

Fevers are typically chronic with drenching night sweats. The patient's blurred vision and red eyes are due to the uveitis. His slurring and facial weakness is secondary to bilateral VII nerve palsy, which usually occurs in Heerfordt's syndrome. Patients often have reduced appetite, as is his being off his food, due to a loss of taste sensation. His swollen face is due to bilateral parotid swelling.

Neurosarcoidosis could cause bilateral VII nerve palsy, fever and blurred vision. Indeed Heerfordt's syndrome involves neurosarcoidosis. However, it is not the answer that would best describe the symptom constellation.

Although anterior uveitis can occur as part of Heerfordt's, it does not account for the other symptoms.

TB is the main red herring here as it could cause all the symptoms described above. However there is nothing in the history to suggest TB infection. Although reactivation of latent TB is associated with immunosuppression, this is typically with anti-TNF-α biologics.

Question 3: Tuberculosis

SBA 1:

Answer: **Lupus pernio**

This rash is pathognomonic of sarcoidosis (it does not occur in other diseases). While Sarcoidosis is the most common cause of erythema nodosum, there are many other conditions associated with it. Maculopapular rashes also occur in sarcoidosis, but this is very non-specific.

Erythema migrans is pathognomonic of Lyme disease. Malar rashes (butterfly rash on the face) most commonly occurs in systemic lupus erythematosus (SLE), but it also occurs in dermatomyositis and pellagra. Neither occurs in sarcoidosis

SBA 2:

Answer: **Short PR interval on ECG**

Sarcoidosis affects the cardiac conduction system classically by presenting with a prolonged, not a shortened, PR interval. Bilateral VII nerve palsy is one of the most common presentations of neurosarcoidosis ($5-10\%$ of sarcoidosis patients will have neurological involvement across the course of their illness). Erythema nodosum is a dermatological manifestation of sarcoidosis. Hepatomegaly in sarcoidosis can be caused by granulomatosis disease in the liver. The parotid glands are commonly involved in sarcoidosis.

SBA 3:

Answer: **Stage I**

Respiratory sarcoidosis is staged I–IV depending on radiological appearance.

Stage 0: No Intrathoracic involvement
Stage I: Bilateral lymphadenopathy
Stage II: Bilateral lymphadenopathy + pulmonary infiltrates
Stage III: Lung parenchymal disease (infiltrates) only
Stage IV: Lung fibrosis

Tuberculosis is endemic in prison populations, especially in Russia and the former Soviet nations. Russian prisons are also frequent sources of MDR-TB and XDR-TB. This man will therefore need to be put in respiratory isolation; he will need PCR and rifampicin probe carried out on his sputum, as well as the routine microscopy and culture.

The calcifications on the chest X-ray suggest cavitations, which are not features of sarcoidosis.

CHAPTER 11: INTERSTITIAL LUNG DISEASE AND VASCULITIS

EMQ:

Answers

Question 1: Dermatomyositis

The patient described is struggling to climb stairs and get out of chairs because of secondary to proximal weakness, which is classical in dermatomyositis, as are generalised symptoms such as fever and weight loss. The aches and pains described are due to the myositis. The purple rash of the face (eyelids) and upper trunk is a heliotrope (purple) rash of the face (eyelids) and upper trunk is typical of dermatomyositis; the rashes on the hands are Gottron's papules. This rash can be worsened by sunlight.

SLE can also present with non-specific symptoms and a photosensitive rash. However, the description of the rash is not typical of SLE. Joint pain is also more typical of SLE than proximal weakness.

Question 2: Idiopathic pulmonary fibrosis.

IPF usually presents at 50–70 years. Having been a farm worker and a smoker are both risk factors for its development, as is a positive family history. Fibrosis is usually in the lower zone of the lungs.

Extrinsic allergic alveolitis is not likely as the symptoms are not sequential to exposure to an allergen and are worsening now that the patient is no longer working on the farm.

Question 3: Drug-induced fibrosis.
The patient's DMARD leflunomide can in rare cases cause pulmonary fibrosis. However, the probable cause of her breathlessness is repeated courses and prolonged use of nitrofurantoin. This can either cause an acute fibrotic reaction, or as in this cause a chronic fibrosis progressing over months or years. The husband and the smoking were distractors.

SBA 1:

Answer: **Anti-Scl 70**
The clinical picture described in this patient is of diffuse scleroderma (DS), as suggested by the lung involvement and the rapid progression of her Raynaud's to sclerosis. Anti-Scl 70 is the only antibody in this list specific for this condition. Her GORD is probably related to oesophageal dysmotility associated with the condition. Autoimmune thyroid disease is associated with this condition.

ACA is associated with limited scleroderma (not the diffuse form), which additionally wouldn't involve the lungs.

Anti-dsDNA is specific for systemic lupus erythematosus.

ANCA is associated with a number of disorders including vasculitides; it has no association with scleroderma.

ANA is a very sensitive test in scleroderma. The use of ANA is very sensitive in scleroderma (+ve - 90−95%), however it is very non-specific and is related with a number of other autoimmune and connective tissue disorders. It would not help in confirming the diagnosis.

SBA 2:

Answer: **B. Bleomycin**
This is the only drug from the list with pulmonary fibrosis as a common recognised side effect.
Vasculitis

SBA 3:

Answer: **1) Eosinophilic granulomatosis with polyangiitis.**
The symptoms described demonstrate the classic prodrome of allergic rhinitis, sinusitis and asthma in teenage years, followed by an eosinophilic and vasculitic pneumonia.

EMQ:

Answers

Question 1: Alpha-1-anti-trypsin deficiency: Many patients are initially diagnosed with asthma, as symptoms are intermittent. The prominent symptoms are wheeze and shortness of breath. Emphysema and dyspnoea develops more than 10 years earlier than in smokers, usually aged 30–45 years. Eventually dyspnoea becomes the prominent symptom. The emphysema causes hyper-expansion of the chest and increased resonance on percussion. Basal emphysema on the chest X-ray is typical in alpha-1-antitrypsin deficiency. Hepatic complications increase with age, many patients develop hepatitis and 15% progress to cirrhosis and liver failure. The deranged LFTs in this patient may suggest hepatic involvement.

Question 2: Idiopathic pulmonary fibrosis. The patient's exposure to dusty environments, due to his job puts him at risk of pulmonary fibrosis. The progressive breathlessness without a cough and the generalised symptoms and malaise are typical of idiopathic pulmonary fibrosis. The fact that both his father and grandfather died of a similar illness would suggest that the patient is part of the 5% that have familial pulmonary fibrosis.

Question 3: Goodpasture's syndrome. The fact that the patient has high blood pressure at such a young age would suggest renal dysfunction. The patient is presenting in his 20s, which would be typical first peak of the bi-modal distribution for Goodpasture's. His smoking also puts him at greater risk of developing Goodpasture's and the haemorrhagic renal and respiratory presentation is typical. The lack of prodromal symptoms as well as the renal involvement makes Churg-Strauss unlikely. The lack of upper respiratory, cutaneous and general manifestations makes Wegner's granulomatosis less likely. It also more typically presents in the 35- to 55-year age range.

SBA 1:

Answer: **Eosinophilic granulomatosis with polyangiitis.** The symptoms described demonstrate the classic prodrome of allergic rhinitis, sinusitis and asthma in teenage years, followed by an eosinophilic and vasculitic pneumonia.

CHAPTER 12: PULMONARY HYPERTENSION

EMQ

Answers

Question 1: Diltiazem. This man has pulmonary hypertension as confirmed and the description suggests that chronic schistosomiasis may be the cause (calcification of the bladder is typical in chronic infection). The diagnosis is confirmed by the right heart catheter. As there is a vasoactive response to the IV epoprostenol, a calcium-channel blocker would be the most appropriate first line treatment.

Question 2: Sildenafil. In reality diuretics, O_2 therapy and anticoagulation would be the initial treatment in this patient, as well as treatment of his hypertension and surgical correction of his stenosis. Calcium channel blockers have no benefit in non-vaso-responsive pulmonary hypertension. The answer to this question is controversial; all of the other pharmacological therapies have a limited evidence base due to the rarity of the disease and NICE has yet to produce guidance on which, if any, is superior. Sildenafil is probably the drug with the most extensive evidence base of symptom improvement. It was the first line drug recommended for WHO group II PH in a consensus statement for physicians in the UK and Ireland published in *Thorax* (http://thorax.bmj.com/content/63/Suppl_2/ii1.full.pdf). However, combination treatment in patients was also recommended.

Question 3: Transplantation (Allogenic)

The patient described has end-stage pulmonary hypertension and. She is deteriorating despite combination medical therapy. She has a congenital patent foramen ovale. The fact that the shunt has reversed and the reversal of the shunt here is a very poor prognostic indicator. Much like in Eisenmenger's syndrome, the fact that the shunt has reversed, as well as the patient not having responded to medical therapy, would indicate that lung transplantation is the only option left.

Atrial balloon septostomy would be of no benefit in this patient as they already have a connection between their two atria.

Xenograft transplantation is not a feasible option: it has never been successfully attempted with a lung.

SBA 1:

Answer: **25 mmHg**

This is the cut off for diagnosing PH. 21–24 mmHg is considered abnormal, however it is borderline and of uncertain clinical significance.

SBA 2:

Answer: **Elevated JVP with a large a wave.**

Pulmonary hypertension causes an elevated JVP with a prominent a wave. If there is eventual tricuspid regurgitation, there may additionally be a large V wave.

Absent x descent is usually seen in atrial fibrillation.

A cannon a wave would indicate ventricular tachycardia, complete heart block or paroxysmal nodal tachycardia.

Kussmaul's sign (paradoxical rise of JVP during inspiration) is typical of cardiac tamponade, but can be seen in right sided cardiac failure. Therefore it may therefore be found in late PH, but would not be a typical finding.

Non-pulsatile elevated JVP would be seen in superior vena caval obstruction.

CHAPTER 13: FUNGAL DISEASES OF THE LUNG

EMQ

Answers

Question 1: Serum LDH: 90% of HIV patients with PCP pneumonia have a raised LDH. Sequential measurements of LDH correlate well with treatment response. Radiological changes only occur weeks after resolution of the illness.

Question 2: VATS + biopsy, culture and staining: This is the gold standard diagnostic test for establishing a diagnosis of invasive broncho-pulmonary aspergillosis, as it gives a tissue diagnosis and has the highest sensitivity and specificity for identification of the organism *Aspergillosis fumigatus*.

Question 3: HIV 1 + 2 antibodies. The patient has been diagnosed with PCP pneumonia. This is an AIDS-defining illness. The patient is new to services and so has not been tested previously. This is likely to be the initial presentation of an HIV infection and the diagnosis needs to be confirmed so that anti-retroviral therapy can be started. PCP pneumonia should not occur in immunocompetent individuals. The microscopy and PAS staining shows clumps resembling crushed "ping pong balls", typical of *P. jirovecii*. The patient has his anti-retrovirals restarted and is put on co-trimoxazole 900 mg OD. What investigation could be done periodically to access treatment response?

SBA 1:

Answer: **15% of cystic fibrosis sufferers have allergic bronchopulmonary aspergillosis. The prevalence is 2% in asthmatics.**

SBA 2:

Answer: **No treatment required. If a mycetoma is asymptomatic, no treatment is required. There is poor evidence for antifungal drugs for the treatment of mycetoma. Surgical treatment should only be considered if there are complications such as haemorrhage or a pneumothorax.**

CHAPTER 14: SLEEP DISORDERED BREATHING

SBA 1:

Answer: **Polysomnography**

This is the gold standard diagnostic test for OSAHS. It measures the number of apnoeic events during a night and can also be used to assess severity.

The Epworth Sleepiness scale score correlates well with OSAHS; however it is not sufficient to make the diagnosis on its own. Nasolaryngoscopy can be used to assess the level of obstruction. Pulse oximetry is not widely used to diagnose OSAHS.

SBA 2:

Answer: **Obesity**

Although all of the above are risk factors for developing OSAHS, having a high BMI is by far the strongest risk factor for developing OSAHS. Losing weight is advocated for treating OSAHS, however as of yet there is only good evidence for this in mild OSAHS.

CHAPTER 15: OCCUPATIONAL LUNG DISEASE

SBA 1:

Answer: **Latex.**

This is a classic history of occupational asthma (plus + allergic dermatitis) caused by latex. This is more common allergen in healthcare workers than chlorhexidine. As a scrub nurse she will be coming into contact with both.

Nothing in the history suggests a food allergy. The dust from the building may aggravate pre-existing asthma if she had a previous history (which she has no history of), and asbestos has a 20–30 year latency period before causing symptoms.

The patient here has no symptoms, but this is likely due to the fact she has been at home over the weekend and away from her working environment over the weekend and has therefore not been in contact with the allergen. She is not malingering; this would be a diagnosis of exclusion after exploring all possible options.

SBA 2:

Answer: **Lifelong smoker**

Smokers who have asbestos-related lung disease are up to 84 times more likely to develop mesothelioma than those who do not. There is limited evidence for the other risk factors increasing risk of mesothelioma, and none has an effect of this magnitude.

CHAPTER 16: RESPIRATORY EMERGENCIES

EMQ: Immediate management of respiratory distress

Question 1

Answer: **Oxygen titrated to ABG results, salbutamol and ipratropium nebs, PO prednisolone.**

This clinical picture and the background history is suggestive of an exacerbation of COPD. Oxygen should be titrated to ABG results due to the risk of CO_2 retention. Nebulisers and steroids (PO or IV should be given).

If there was evidence of infection, you should also start oral antibiotics.

Question 2

Answer: **15L O_2 via non re-breathe mask, IM adrenaline, IV hydrocortisone**

Shortness of breath and wheeze in a patient of this age may suggest asthma, but the facial swelling raises suspicion of anaphylaxis, especially if she gives a history of exposure to a known allergen. Immediate treatment should be according to the ABCDE approach along with adrenaline and IV steroids.

Question 3

Answer: **Urgent needle decompression**

This clinical picture is suggestive of a left sided pneumothorax. Urgent needle decompression is required, followed by insertion of a chest drain.

SBAs

Question 1

Answer: **High-dose dexamethasone.**

The clinical picture is suggestive of superior vena cava obstruction, causing venous congestion in the face and arms. The immediate management of this is high dose dexamethasone (with PPI cover). Referral for SVC stenting can be considered in this situation. You should identify and treat the underlying cause.

CHAPTER 17: SMOKING AND THE LUNG

SBA 1:

Answer: **15%**

Only a small minority of patients who use the NHS stop smoking service are still abstinent at 1 year, compared to 4% of people who attempt to stop without help.

A short-term quit rate of up to 25% is reported with nicotine replacement therapy combined with counselling.

SBA 2:

Answer: **32-year-old woman smokes 20 cigarettes a day and expresses a wish to quit smoking. She had asthma as a child but otherwise has no PMH and is fit and well. She admits to needing counselling and treatment previously for self-harming.**

The patient has a history of what could possibly be serious mental health issues. This is an absolute contraindication for prescribing varenicline.

Courses of varenicline can be continued for a further 12 weeks after completion of initial course, at the discretion of the clinician.

Previous seizures (especially one off events in childhood) are not a contraindication. If a patient had a current seizure disorder the use of varenicline use would be cautioned but not completely contraindicated.

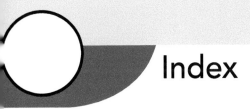

Index

Note: Page numbers in *italics* indicate a figure and page numbers in **bold** indicate a table on the corresponding page.